Psychosis in Adolescents and Adults with Intellectual Disabilities

Trine Lise Bakken
Editor

Psychosis in Adolescents and Adults with Intellectual Disabilities

New Knowledge and Clinical Implications

palgrave
macmillan

Editor
Trine Lise Bakken
Oslo University Hospital
Oslo, Norway

ISBN 978-3-031-95317-0 ISBN 978-3-031-95318-7 (eBook)
https://doi.org/10.1007/978-3-031-95318-7

This Palgrave Macmillan imprint is published by the registered company Springer Nature Switzerland AG
The registered company address is: Gewerbestrasse 11, 6330 Cham, Switzerland

I dedicate this book to the patients with psychosis I have met, through the more than forty years in mental health services.

Preface I

My first experience with psychosis was reading the famous book written by Fyodor Dostoyevsky, *The double*, at the age of 16. At 19, in January 1978, I started as a nurse assistant in a mental health inpatient unit for elderly women with schizophrenia. One of the patients was 84 at that time. We developed a good relationship through frequent conversations and solving crossword puzzles together. I visited her often after quitting after 6 months, during five years until she passed away. When we first met, she told me that her oesophagus was only one millimetre wide; hence she could not eat normal food. I knew only very little about anatomy. I believed what she told me, and made orange juice and thin soups for her. The head nurse came to know about my cooking activities. I was summoned, and given a reprimand. I was told that the patient was delusional. I have carried this experience with me ever since, respecting that delusional ideas appear as real to the patient.

Since then, schizophrenia has been my main field of interest in mental health services. Firstly, in general mental health services, predominantly in acute wards. For the last thirty years, I have worked in a regional specialised department for patients with ID and mental disorders, at the Oslo University Hospital. I have had the possibility to participate in research, beside clinical work.

Trine Lise Bakken
National Advisory Unit for
Mental Health in Intellectual
Disabilities
Oslo University Hospital
Oslo, Norway

Preface II

The work with this book started with an invitation from the Publisher Palgrave Macmillan. I met one of the editors, Clelia Petracca, at the EAMHID, European Association of Mental Health in Intellectual Disability, conference in Helsinki in September 2023. A book proposal on psychosis in intellectual disability was accepted, and then this book was planned. I invited colleges from Demark, Norway, and Italy to contribute on specialist topics, which is outside my area of expertise: developmental psychology, biological medicine, and occupational therapy. Many thanks to Charlotte Andersen (Denmark), Kjersti Karlsen, (Norway) Jacopo Santambrogi and Emma Francia, both Italy. The content of the book is addressed in the introduction, which is Chapter 1. There has been no funding of this book.

Asker, Norway — Trine Lise Bakken

Acknowledgements

Without support and encouragement from professors in psychiatry, psychology, and nursing, this book would not have been written. When I first started to look into the phenomenology of schizophrenia in patients with intellectual disability, there was only minimal academic or clinical interest in severe mental illness in persons with ID in Norway. However, when I met Anton Dosen at a conference in Berlin in 2001, he was the first to take an interest in my vague ideas of how to investigate psychotic symptoms in people who sparsely speak. Since then, my Norwegian supervisors, professor Nina Smeby, professor Svein Friis, and professor Harald Martinsen have all supported my research. Thank you all! Thanks also to psychiatrist Sverre Løvoll, who had to listen to me and discuss this topic from 1995 and for two decades.

Contents

Contributors

Charlotte Andersen Fredericia, Denmark

Trine Lise Bakken Oslo University Hospital, Oslo, Norway

Emma Francia Milan, Italy

Kjersti Karlsen Oslo University Hospital, Oslo, Norway

Jacopo Santambrogio Azienda Socio Sanitaria Territoriale della Brianza, Limbiate, Italy

Abbreviations

ASD	Autism Spectrum Disorders
BtC	Behaviour that Challenges
ID	Intellectual Disability

1

Introduction

Trine Lise Bakken

Abstract This chapter presents an overview of the historical aspects of psychosis in intellectual disabilities. Additionally, the current knowledge about prevalence, age of onset, symptoms, and prognosis. Aetiology is included in the chapter about biological aspects. From the late 1800s, severe mental health conditions and "mental retardation" (now intellectual disabilities) were seen as closely connected, which is reflected in the International Classification of Diseases, ICD, in which both mental health conditions and intellectual disabilities, including neurodevelopmental disorders, up until the last decades have been placed in the same chapter. In this book, the current diagnostic subgroups of psychosis will not be presented or discussed. Psychosis in bipolar disorder and major depression will not be presented or discussed. This book emphasizes phenomenology, diagnostics, biological aspects, interventions and treatment, and user' and their family's experiences.

T. L. Bakken (✉)
Oslo University Hospital, Oslo, Norway
e-mail: uxtlba@ous-hf.no

T. L. Bakken (ed.), *Psychosis in Adolescents and Adults with Intellectual Disabilities*,
https://doi.org/10.1007/978-3-031-95318-7_1

Keywords Psychosis · Prevalence · Onset · Co-morbidity · Genetic syndromes

History

Historically, mental health conditions in people with intellectual disabilities have not been adequately addressed. People with intellectual disabilities and psychosis have often "fallen between" the specialized mental health services for the general population and the specialized services for people with intellectual disabilities (Bakken & Sageng, 2016). Before the 1990s, most people with intellectual disabilities in the Western hemisphere spent their adult lives in specialized institutions for people with intellectual disabilities (Bredewold et al., 2020; Nøttestad & Linaker, 2001). During the deinstitutionalization era, it became evident that people with intellectual disabilities also suffer from mental health conditions. The ideal has been that people with intellectual disabilities should benefit from general psychiatric services when experiencing mental health problems (Chowdhury & Benson, 2011). However, it is argued that the main challenge for professionals dealing with mental health conditions in people with intellectual disabilities is not the organization of services (general or specialized, inpatient or ambulatory), but the competence, or lack thereof, of the caring staff (Bakken & Sageng, 2016; Hall et al., 2006). General mental health services often lack knowledge about the unique challenges of assessing and treating mental health conditions in people with intellectual disabilities (Chaplin, 2009; Lunsky et al., 2010). Despite progress in the field, including increased knowledge and research, people with intellectual disabilities still face barriers when seeking access to mental health services.

It has previously been assumed that psychosis could not occur in people with an IQ lower than approximately 50, who cannot report on core features (Reid, 1972). It has also been claimed that psychosis cannot be diagnosed in "idiots" (Reid, 1972). Nevertheless, psychosis in people with intellectual disabilities has been described already in the late nineteenth century (Reid, 1972). Most of the knowledge about psychosis in people with intellectual disabilities is from studies involving people with mild intellectual disabilities.

Regarding people with both intellectual disabilities and autism spectrum disorder, it was previously believed that psychosis did not occur in people with autism, a view reflected in earlier diagnostic criteria. The co-occurrence of autism and psychosis was first acknowledged in the diagnostic manuals ICD-10 and DSM-IV, released in 1993/1994.

Until about year 2000, there was a dearth of studies on how symptoms in people with more severe intellectual disabilities manifest. Adults with intellectual disabilities and psychosis may during episodes of psychosis appear severely disturbed (Bakken, 2014; Cherry et al., 2000). They display disorientation, disorganized behaviour, and agitation or aggression. Even in those with mild intellectual disabilities, their language skills severely deteriorate (Bakken et al., 2023). They are more or less unavailable for social contact and display severely reduced global functioning. Thus, the person has considerable problems with task performance, social interaction and basic self-care (Bakken et al., 2024). Due to impaired ability to report their symptoms, they have an increased chance of their mental illness being overseen. This is also the fact for those with mild intellectual disabilities. Since their actions appear chaotic, both professional and informal caregivers will for the most part, not understand what the person tries to communicate, which may impair the caregiver's ability to respond therapeutically. Research after year 2000 underpins the total burden of signs and symptoms of severe mental health conditions as higher in the whole group of people with intellectual disabilities—from mild to profound degree (Gustafsson & Sonnander, 2004). It has been suggested that this might be explained by initially weaker reality testing. It has also been suggested that people with intellectual disabilities and psychoses tend to need more time to gain pre-psychotic functioning, compared to the general population (Bakken et al., 2024).

Prevalence

Research has shown that people with intellectual disabilities are at a higher risk of developing mental health conditions compared to those in the general population (Bakken, et al., 2024; Cooper et al., 2007). The lifetime prevalence of psychosis in the general population is estimated to be about 0.5% (Saha et al., 2005; Simeone et al., 2015). Though there is considerable variation in methodologies, settings, and sample sizes in studies of psychosis in people with intellectual disabilities, the prevalence has been found to be at least tripled compared to the general population (Cooper et al., 2007).

In a recent Swedish register study including all people living in Skaane, in the south of Sweden, about 1,250,000 people, the prevalence of psychosis in the general population was about 0.9% (Bakken et al. 2024). In the Skaane population, about 15,000 people were diagnosed with intellectual disabilities. Among them, the overall prevalence of diagnoses in the psychosis spectrum (F20–29) was 7.2%, about eight times higher than in the general population. However, the relative risk (RR) of psychosis was about 15 in those with mild intellectual disabilities versus the general population. The RR was about 13 in those with moderate intellectual disabilities versus the general population, and about 4 in those with severe or profound intellectual disabilities (Bakken et al., 2024). It is still not proven if these large differences in relative risk are due to real numbers or if they are due to diagnostic overshadowing—that people with more severe difficulties in reporting symptoms of mental health conditions are given other explanations for their difficulties.

People with autism spectrum disorder (ASD) have been reported to have a high risk for co-occurring psychosis (Vaquerizo-Serrano et al., 2022). However, there are clear diagnostic limitations for the group of people with limited communication abilities with ASD with additional ID. This requires a critical reflection on the presumed frequencies. In the Swedish population study, the results indicated no increased risk of being diagnosed with a condition on the psychosis spectrum for those with both ID and ASD, compared to those with ID and no ASD diagnosis (Bakken et al., 2024).

The prevalence of psychosis in people with intellectual disabilities in clinical settings is found to be very high. In a Norwegian clinical study, 26 of 183 participants in specialized mental health services for people with intellectual disabilities, or in adult habilitation services, were diagnosed with psychosis in the schizophrenia spectrum. A cross-sectional study conducted in a clinical sample of 120 persons with ID and comorbid mental health conditions in three Italian residential facilities, using SPAIDD-G tools to assess diagnostic orientations of mental health conditions, found a prevalence of 38% (46 persons) (Santambrogio et al., 2023).

Onset and Prognosis

It has been assumed that the age of onset of psychosis is significantly lower in people with intellectual disabilities compared to the general population. However, knowledge about the onset of conditions in the psychosis spectrum in people with intellectual disabilities is sparse. Despite assumptions about early or very early onset, often referred to as childhood onset of psychosis, in people with intellectual disabilities (Jolly et al., 2013), there are limited data. A French study, which included a large clinical sample of about 700 consecutively recruited people diagnosed with psychosis, compared people with adult-onset psychosis to those with childhood-onset psychosis (Coulon et al., 2020). The group with childhood-onset psychosis had significantly lower educational levels and more frequently a history of learning impairments. In the Swedish population study mentioned above, it was found that among children, the risk of having a diagnosis in the psychosis spectrum was more than nine times higher than among children in the general population (Bakken et al., 2024). This is a crucial finding, as it supports earlier assumptions that the onset of psychosis is significantly earlier in people with intellectual disabilities. The clinical implications suggest that child mental health services and child habilitation services must consider the possibility that severe global declines in functioning, and also behavioural changes, may be symptoms of psychosis.

The long-term outcome of psychosis is heterogeneous, ranging from full remission to severe chronic conditions (Volavka & Vevera, 2018). A review study found that psychosis had worse outcomes compared to other diagnostic groups such as schizoaffective or affective conditions (Lang et al., 2013). Lang and colleagues found that psychopathological symptoms remained relatively stable over the course of the illness. Several predictors for a poor outcome were identified, such as male gender and a high symptom load of negative symptoms.

Both prognosis and the course of psychosis are generally understudied in people with intellectual disabilities. In a Norwegian clinical study, a group of 26 autistic adolescents with intellectual disabilities diagnosed with schizophrenic psychosis, participated in a multicentre study on mental health in people with intellectual disabilities, and co-occurring autism spectrum disorder (Bakken et al., 2024). The scores at discharge indicated that multimodal treatment of co-occurring psychosis appears feasible and effective in people with intellectual disabilities. At 1-year follow-up, the scores were still indicating the same treatment effects as at discharge.

Co-occurrence of Genetic Syndromes

Genetic syndromes are known to be associated with psychosis in the general population (Singh et al., 2017). The syndrome most closely associated with psychosis is 22q11 Deletion Syndrome, also known as Di George syndrome (Patel et al., 2022). Other chromosomal abnormalities, such as Klinefelter syndrome and Turner syndrome, are also associated with an increased risk of psychosis (Cederlöf et al., 2014; Prior et al., 2000). Contrary to earlier assumptions of a low risk of psychosis in people with Down syndrome, Dykens et al. (2015) found an increased risk of psychosis in people with Down syndrome compared to other people with intellectual disabilities. Regarding Fragile X syndrome, an American comparative study found that the use of anti-psychotic medication was more than four times higher in people with Fragile X syndrome compared to the general population (Nazaret et al., 2016).

Co-morbidity

People with intellectual disabilities are at higher risk of developing co-morbid mental health conditions compared to the general population (Cooper et al., 2007). Specifically, a Swedish register study found that people diagnosed with both intellectual disabilities and psychosis had a significantly higher risk of developing co-morbid mental health conditions compared to those with only intellectual disabilities or only psychosis (Bakken, Axmon & Sandberg, submitted). Also, physical conditions are more frequently present in people with psychosis (Kugathasan et al., 2019), and in people with intellectual disabilities (Glover et al., 2017). More about co-morbidity of physical conditions in Chapter 6.

Access to Services

The problems of limited access to mental health assessment, treatment and care arose after the phasing down of the centralized institutions in for people with intellectual disabilities who have multiple and complex needs (Nøttestad & Linaker, 2001). The multidisciplinary teams that worked in the larger institutions were broken up. The community-based programmes resulted in fragmentation of services (Gibbs & Priest, 1999; Graham, 2004). This is a less than satisfactory situation for the most vulnerable users, especially those with complex multiple needs. A Dutch study found services in the communities deteriorated for the most vulnerable people with disabilities after the deinstitutionalization of services (Bredewold et al., 2020). Bredewold and colleagues ask whether the deinstitutionalization has led to real inclusion in society. Furthermore, they ask whether community services, mainly in group homes, really is cheaper than large-scale institutional care that has for the most part been abandoned in Western Europe.

Interventions and Treatment

Interventions and treatment are still sparsely studied. Recommended interventions and treatment for people with intellectual disabilities, diagnosed with psychosis, should follow a bio-psycho-social approach, often referred to as "combination therapy," encompassing medication, psychosocial interventions, and community services. The research literature, however, for the most part, addresses treatment with psychopharmacologic medication, and psychosocial interventions based on interventions for the general population (Chisholm et al., 2016; Humphries et al., 2020). Most studies present case studies or studies with a limited number of participants. Gold standard studies with randomized, controlled, representative samples are still ahead for this group.

Core Terms

Intellectual disabilities: the diagnostic term for intellectual disabilities was previously "mental retardation" in DSM-IV and ICD-10 (APA, 1994; WHO, 1992), but this term was infrequently used in clinical practice and research. The term "intellectual disabilities" is currently in use, although the diagnostic criteria are "Disorder of Intellectual Development" in ICD-11 and "Intellectual Developmental Disorder" in DSM-5 (APA, 2013). This book uses the term "intellectual disabilities."

Psychosis is a term used to describe severe mental health conditions characterized by a loss of contact with reality. The root of the term, "psyche," is from Greek, meaning "mind" or "soul," while "osis" is Latin and means "abnormal condition." In this book, the term "psychosis" includes psychosis in the schizophrenia spectrum (ICD-11). The severe mental health conditions, bipolar disorder, and major depression with psychotic symptoms will not be addressed.

The term **autism** was first introduced by child psychiatrist Kanner (1943). "Autism" (from Greek "auto" = self) originally referred to the schizophrenic symptom of extreme social withdrawal. Although the condition has long been differentiated from the psychosis spectrum (Fish & Rivto, 1979), the term has persisted.

It should be noted that people with intellectual disabilities constitute a largely heterogeneous group; ranging from people with borderline IQ and only minor problems associated with having intellectual disabilities, to users with more severe intellectual disabilities, and additional neurocognitive disorders; the most severe being autism spectrum disorder. Also, mental health conditions, vision and/or hearing impairments, dysfunctional sensory processing, and physical conditions are more frequently occurring in people with intellectual disabilities, compared to the general population. The latter constitutes a subgroup of people with intellectual disabilities and multiple complex needs (Bakken & Ellingsen, 2024; Cook & Hole, 2021). In people with intellectual disabilities, who have multiple, complex needs, stress is found to occur frequently (Scott & Havercamp, 2014), and stress is associated with behaviour that challenges (BtC). People with severe mental health conditions addition to intellectual disabilities, especially those with moderate—severe grade, and additional neurocognitive conditions, usually have multiple, complex needs, and hence may show BtC, which may overshadow the mental health condition.

People with intellectual disabilities who have multiple, complex needs may have problems with both introspection and spoken language due to their low intellectual functioning and additional conditions such as autism, mental health, physical conditions, and sensory loss (Bakken et al., 2023; Doodeman et al., 2022).

This is also the case for those with mild intellectual disabilities. The lack of introspection and mentalizing abilities, addition to psychotic symptoms, may cause insurmountable challenges regarding the reporting of inner representations, especially delusions and hallucinations. Hence, also in those with mild intellectual disabilities, the use of observable symptoms may be necessary.

The Chosen Topics in This Book

The topics chosen for this book are based on available research and 30 years of clinical experience in this field, as well as collaborations with colleagues both internationally and in Norway.

Phenomenology, the appearance of symptoms, is a key topic, as understanding symptoms is crucial for both assessment and treatment (Chapter 2). This is particularly important because psychotic symptoms and behaviours can easily be mistaken for challenging behaviour, especially during acute phases. The chapter on assessment (Chapter 3) references research and presents useful tools. Current recommendations for assessing psychosis in people with intellectual disabilities include a multimodal approach conducted by multidisciplinary teams. Assessing mental health conditions involves not only identifying the most appropriate diagnoses but also excluding other possible diagnoses. Many mental and physical conditions can be mistaken for psychosis in people with intellectual disabilities (Chapter 4). Recent research highlights the importance of emotional development in people with intellectual disabilities for providing adequate services. Emotional development is often found to be delayed in people with intellectual disabilities who also have mental health conditions. The measurement of adaptive skills may follow a similar pattern to emotional development. Assessing levels of emotional development and adaptive skills can provide valuable information for treatment and care (Chapter 5).

Research over the past two decades has provided new insights into the biological aspects of psychosis, which also inform psychopharmacological treatment (Chapter 6). Combination therapy is recommended for treating psychosis in people with intellectual disabilities. Psychosocial interventions include various individual and group treatments, adapted for people with intellectual disabilities (Chapter 7). Sensory therapy has been shown to provide symptom relief (Chapter 8).

Although there are no representative studies on user or family experiences, existing studies emphasize the importance of a strong working alliance for people with intellectual disabilities who are provided mental health services (Chapter 9).

Conclusive Remarks

The history of mental health in people with intellectual disabilities is relatively short, particularly in acknowledging that people in this group can have mental health conditions. Research in this area began in the 1970s but gained significant momentum after the year 2000, and it is still in its infancy. Most assessments, treatments, and interventions are adapted from those developed for the general population, reflecting the view that mental health conditions are similar across both groups. However, research on outcomes for people with intellectual disabilities is mostly not at the highest level, such as randomized controlled trials (RCTs).

References

American Psychiatric Association, APA. (1994). DSM-IV. *Diagnostic and statistical manual of mental disorders* (4th ed.). American Psychiatric Association.

American Psychiatric Association, APA. (2013). DSM-V. *Diagnostic and statistical manual of mental disorders* (5th ed.). American Psychiatric Association.

Bakken, T. L. (2014). Psychosis and disorganized behaviour in adults with autism and intellectual disability: Case identification and staff-patient interaction. In V. B. Patel, V. Preedy, & C. R. Martin (Eds.), *Comprehensive guide to autism* (pp. 585–600). Springer Science.

Bakken, T. L., Askeland Hellerud, J. M., Kildahl, A. N., Solheim-Inderberg, A. M., Helverschou, S. B., & Hove, O. (2024). Psychosis in autistic people with intellectual disabilities. Treatment and interventions. *Journal of Autism and Developmental Disorders,* 1–11.

Bakken, T. L., & Ellingsen, B. (2024). The effects of lockdown of work and activities for adults with multiple, complex needs including sensory impairments during the pandemic in 2020. *Journal of Intellectual Disabilities.* https://doi.org/10.1177/17446295241232030

Bakken, T. L., Kildahl, A. N., Ludvigsen, L. B., Bjørgen, T. G., Dalhaug, C., Hellerud, J. M. A., Hove, O., Solheim-Inderberg, A. M., Karlsen, K., & Helverschou, S. B. (2023). Psychosis in autistic people with intellectual disabilities: Symptom manifestations and identification. *Journal of Applied Research in Intellectual Disabilities.*

Bakken, T. L., & Sageng, H. (2016). Mental health nursing of adults with intellectual disabilities and mental illness: A review of empirical studies 1994–2013. *Archives of Psychiatric Nursing, 30*(2), 286–291.

Bredewold, F., Hermus, M., & Trappenburg, M. (2020). Living in the community' the pros and cons: A systematic literature review of the impact of deinstitutionalisation on people with intellectual and psychiatric disabilities. *Journal of Social Work, 20*(1), 83–116.

Cederlöf, M., Gotby, A. O., Larsson, H., Serlachius, E., Boman, M., Långström, N., Landén, M., & Lichtenstein, P. (2014). Klinefelter syndrome and risk of psychosis, autism and ADHD. *Journal of Psychiatric Research, 48*(1), 128–130.

Chaplin, R. (2009). Annotation: New research into general psychiatric services for adults with intellectual disability and mental illness. *Journal of Intellectual Disability Research, 53*(3), 189–199.

Cherry, K. E., Penn, D., Matson, J. L., & Bamburg, J. W. (2000). Characteristics of psychosis among persons with severe or profound mental retardation. *Psychiatric Services, 51*(7), 922–924.

Chisholm, K., Lin, A., & Armando, M. (2016). Psychosis spectrum disorders and autism spectrum disorder. In *Psychiatric symptoms and comorbidities in autism spectrum disorder* (pp. 51–66).

Chowdhury, M., & Benson, B. A. (2011). Deinstitutionalization and quality of life of individuals with intellectual disability: A review of the international literature. *Journal of Policy and Practice in Intellectual Disability, 8*(4), 256–265.

Cook, S., & Hole, R. (2021). Trauma, intellectual and/or developmental disability, and multiple, complex needs: A scoping review of the literature. *Research in Developmental Disabilities, 115*, Article 103939.

Cooper, S. A., Smiley, E., Morrison, J., Williamson, A., & Allan, L. (2007). Mental ill-health in adults with intellectual disabilities: Prevalence and associated factors. *The British Journal of Psychiatry, 190*(1), 27–35.

Coulon, N., Godin, O., Bulzacka, E., Dubertret, C., Mallet, J., Fond, G., Brunel, L., Andrianarisoa, M., Anderson, G., Chereau, I., Denizot, H., Rey, R., Dorey, J. M., Lançon, C., Faget, C., Roux, P., Passerieux, C., Dubreucq, J., Leignier, S., ... Schürhoff, F. (2020). Early and very early-onset psychosis compared with adult-onset psychosis: French FACE-SZ database. *Brain and Behavior, 10*(2), e01495.

Doodeman, T. W., Schuengel, C., & Sterkenburg, P. S. (2022). Expressions of stress of people with severe intellectual disabilities and sensitive caregiving to regulate stress: A qualitative study. *Journal of Intellectual & Developmental Disability, 47*(4), 308–317.

Dykens, E. M., Shah, B., Davis, B., Baker, C., Fife, T., & Fitzpatrick, J. (2015). Psychiatric disorders in adolescents and young adults with Down syndrome and other intellectual disabilities. *Journal of Neurodevelopmental Disorders, 7*(1), 1–8.

Fish, B., & Rivto, E. R. (1979). Psychosis of childhood. In J. D. Noshpitzs (Ed.), *Basic handbook of child psychiatry* (Vol. 2, pp. 249–303). Basic Books.

Gibbs, M., & Priest, H. M. (1999). Designing and implementing a 'dual diagnosis' module: A review of the literature and some preliminary findings. *Nurse Education Today, 19*, 357–363.

Glover, G., Williams, R., Heslop, P., Oyinlola, J., & Grey, J. (2017). Mortality in people with intellectual disabilities in England. *Journal of Intellectual Disability Research, 61*(1), 62–74.

Graham, J. (2004). Communicating with the uncommunicative: Music therapy with pre-verbal adults. *British Journal of Learning Disabilities, 32*(1), 24–33.

Gustafsson, C., & Sonnander, K. (2004). Occurrence of mental health problems in Swedish samples of adults with intellectual disabilities. *Social Psychiatry and Psychiatric Epidemiology, 39*, 448–456.

Hall, I., Parkes, C., Samuels, S., & Hassiotis, A. (2006). Working across boundaries: Clinical outcomes for an integrated mental health service for people with intellectual disabilities. *Journal of Intellectual Disability Research, 50*(8), 598–607.

Humphries, L., Michael, D., & Hassiotis, A. (2020). Psychosis and related psychoses in people with intellectual disability. In *Oxford textbook of the psychiatry of intellectual disability* (pp. 91–104).

Jolly, L. A., Homan, C. C., Jacob, R., Barry, S., & Gecz, J. (2013). The UPF3B gene, implicated in intellectual disability, autism, ADHD and childhood onset psychosis regulates neural progenitor cell behaviour and neuronal outgrowth. *Human Molecular Genetics, 22*(23), 4673–4687.

Kanner, L. (1943). Autistic disturbances of affective contact. *Journal of Nervous Child, 2*, 217–250.

Kugathasan, P., Stubbs, B., Aagaard, J., Jensen, S. E., Munk Laursen, T., & Nielsen, R. E. (2019). Increased mortality from somatic multimorbidity in patients with psychosis: A Danish nationwide cohort study. *Acta Psychiatrica Scandinavica, 140*(4), 340–348.

Lang, F. U., Koesters, M., Lang, S., Becker, T., & Jaeger, M. (2013). Psychopathological long-term outcome of psychosis—A review. *Acta Psychiatrica Scandinavica, 127*(3), 173–182.

Lunsky, Y., White, S. E., Palucka, A. M., Weiss, J., Bockus, S., & Gofine, T. (2010). Clinical outcomes of a specialised inpatient unit for adults with mild to severe intellectual disability and mental illness. *Journal of Intellectual Disability Research, 54*(1), 60–69.

Nazareth, T., Li, N., Marynchenko, M., Zhou, Z., Chopra, P., Signorovitch, J., et al. (2016). Burden of illness among patients with fragile X syndrome (FXS): A Medicaid perspective. *Current Medical Research and Opinion, 32*(3), 405–416.

Nøttestad, J. A., & Linaker, O. M. (2001). Self-injurious behaviour before and after deinstitutionalization. *Journal of Intellectual Disability Research, 45*(2), 121–129.

Patel, H., Vadukapuram, R., Mansuri, Z., Trivedi, C., Brar, K. S., & Beg, U. (2022). Psychiatric comorbidities in adults with DiGeorge syndrome. *Clinical Psychopharmacology and Neuroscience, 20*(3), 498.

Prior, T. I., Chue, P. S., & Tibbo, P. (2000). Investigation of Turner syndrome in psychosis. *American Journal of Medical Genetics, 96*(3), 373–378.

Reid, A. H. (1972). Psychoses in adult mental defectives: II. Schizophrenic and paranoid psychoses. *British Journal of Psychiatry, 120*, 213–218.

Saha, S., Chant, D., Welham, J., & McGrath, J. (2005). A systematic review of the prevalence of psychosis. *PLoS Medicine, 2*(5), Article e141.

Santambrogio, J., Bertelli, M. O., Terrevazzi, S., De Carolis, L., Francia, E., Boldoni, C., Calascibetta, M., Cudazzo, E., Lucca, C., Viganò, V., Danese, M., Minazzi, G. A., Santarone, A., Bianco, A., Hassiotis, A., & Clerici, M. (2023). Cognitive dysfunction and psychopathology: A cohort study of adults with intellectual developmental disorder. *Journal of Intellectual Disability Research, 67*(10), 1029–1045.

Scott, H. M., & Havercamp, S. M. (2014). Mental health for people with intellectual disability: The impact of stress and social support. *American Journal on Intellectual and Developmental Disabilities, 119*(6), 552–564.

Simeone, J. C., Ward, A. J., Rotella, P., Collins, J., & Windisch, R. (2015). An evaluation of variation in published estimates of psychosis prevalence from 1990–2013: A systematic literature review. *BMC Psychiatry, 15*(1), 1–14.

Singh, T., Walters, J. T., Johnstone, M., Curtis, D., Suvisaari, J., Torniainen, M., Rees, E., Iyegbe, C., Blackwood, D., McIntosh, A. M., Kirov, G., Geschwind, D., Murray, R. M., Di Forti, M., Bramon, E., Gandal, M., Hultman, C. M., Sklar, P., INTERVAL Study, … Barrett, J. C. (2017). The contribution of rare variants to risk of psychosis in individuals with and without intellectual disability. *Nature Genetics, 49*(8), 1167–1173

Vaquerizo-Serrano, J., de Pablo, S. D., Singh, J., & Santosh, P. (2022). Autism spectrum disorder and clinical high risk for psychosis: A systematic review and meta-analysis. *Journal of Autism and Developmental Disorders, 52*(4), 568–1586.

Volavka, J., & Vevera, J. (2018). Very long-term outcome of psychosis. *International Journal of Clinical Practice, 72*(7), Article e13094.

World Health Organization. (1992). *The ICD-10 classification of mental and behavioural disorders: Clinical descriptions and diagnostic guidelines*. World Health Organization.

2

Psychotic Symptoms in People with Intellectual Disabilities

Trine Lise Bakken

Abstract Understanding symptoms is crucial for both diagnostic assessment and treatment. Using conventional criteria to assess psychosis in people with intellectual disabilities can be challenging due to communication difficulties and because language deterioration is a hallmark of psychosis. In general, the same symptoms may appear in various mental health conditions. For people with limited ability to report their inner states or symptoms, observing behavioural equivalents may be a solution. The risk of misattributing symptoms, such as interpreting idiosyncratic beliefs and behaviours in people with intellectual disabilities as delusions, is addressed in the chapter on differential diagnostics.

Keywords Psychotic symptoms · Delusions · Hallucinations · Disorganization · Negative symptoms · Prodromal symptoms · Observable symptoms

T. L. Bakken (✉)
Oslo University Hospital, Oslo, Norway
e-mail: uxtlba@ous-hf.no

T. L. Bakken (ed.), *Psychosis in Adolescents and Adults with Intellectual Disabilities*,
https://doi.org/10.1007/978-3-031-95318-7_2

Premorbid Symptoms

Self-disturbances are core phenotypical features of psychosis (Baklund et al., 2024), also known as anomalous self-experiences or self-disorder. These disturbances are considered a hallmark of schizophrenic psychosis, distinguishing it from other psychotic conditions such as bipolar disorder. Premorbid self-disorders (also called prodromal schizophrenic symptoms) include alienating experiences, ephemerality, and identity diffuseness (Parnas et al., 2016). Symptoms described include immense feelings of being different from peers and not finding a place in the world, which has been documented in psychosis literature for decades (Heinimaa et al., 2003).

Premorbid functioning is scarcely studied in people with intellectual disabilities who are later diagnosed with psychosis. A few case studies present symptoms in people with psychosis and additional intellectual disabilities or autism spectrum disorder (e.g., Bakken & Høidal, 2014; Bakken et al., 2009). A study published in 2004 describes early onset psychosis in 21 adolescents with intellectual disabilities (<18 years), presenting both typical and atypical symptoms, but no typical prodromal symptoms are described (Friedlander & Donnelly, 2004). However, for those with concurrent autism spectrum disorder and intellectual disabilities, clinicians should be aware of the similarities between self-disturbances in psychosis and autism spectrum disorder (Noel et al., 2017). Both groups are found to have a weak sense of self and identity issues. Despite these similarities, Noel and colleagues argue that there is one significant difference: the way people interact with others (2017). While people with autism spectrum disorder have sharper boundaries between self and others, those with psychosis tend to show more blurred self-other boundaries.

Delusions, Hallucinations, Disorganization, and Negative Symptoms

Like people in the general population, people with intellectual disabilities who are diagnosed with psychosis may appear disorganized and severely disturbed during acute phases or periods of high symptom load (Bakken, 2021; Bakken et al., 2007; WHO, 2018). Clinical studies have found that people with intellectual disabilities display similarly fragmented speech and behavioural patterns as those observed in the general population during acute phases of psychosis (Bakken & Høidal, 2014; Bakken et al., 2009). However, for practitioners unfamiliar with a person suspected of having psychosis, these speech and behavioural patterns may be challenging to distinguish from difficulties associated with intellectual disabilities. To make an adequate differentiation, obtaining a thorough developmental history, including information about potential symptom trajectories, is essential (Siegel et al., 2020).

Delusions are commonly described as strange beliefs not shared by others, often involving paranoid ideas about being watched or that others have evil intentions (WHO, 2018). Most people in the general population can report delusions. However, people with intellectual disabilities, even those with borderline intellectual functioning or mild intellectual disabilities, may become non-verbal during episodes of acute psychosis (Bakken et al., 2007; Engebretsen et al., 2019). Those with additional autism spectrum disorder may have aggravated difficulties reporting delusions and hallucinations due to decreased introspection and poor abilities of mentalisation (Robinson et al., 2017). Consequently, they may not recognize what is unusual to experience and tend not to report strange beliefs (Bakken et al., 2009). However, people with mild or moderate intellectual disabilities will usually report delusions at least once the acute phase is in remission (Bakken et al., 2007).

Hallucinations, described as deceptions of the senses, can occur in all sensory modalities: sight, hearing, smell, and touch. Observable symptoms of hallucinations in people with intellectual disabilities are often referred to as "suspected hallucinations" and "pseudopsychotic symptoms" (Bakken et al., 2007; Hurley, 2003). Signs of hallucinations described by Bakken et al. (2007) and Hurley (2003) include "staring at fixed points and yelling, covering ears while making strange sounds, earaches without otitis, talking to oneself out loud, talking to people who are not there, talking out loud when upset, experiencing unexplainable sensations, and saying they see things that are not there." In both studies, most participants had mild or moderate intellectual disabilities and typically possessed verbal abilities.

Disorganization is one of the main symptoms of psychosis. It is observable and therefore of special interest for investigating people with intellectual disabilities who are suspected of being psychotic. A Norwegian case study examined the co-occurrence of speech and behavioural disorganization in an adult with psychosis and mild intellectual disabilities (Bakken et al., 2009). The presence of disorganized speech and behaviour was rated by two experienced mental health nurse specialists, through observations of videotaped user-staff interactions. The strong relationship between disorganized speech and behaviour generates a hypothesis of a general concurrence of the two. Valid behavioural indicators will facilitate the recognition of schizophrenia in people with limited verbal skills, as well as introspective abilities.

Negative symptoms, such as fatigue, lack of motivation, and social withdrawal, may be observed as behavioural equivalents at all levels of intellectual disabilities. Aggravated social withdrawal is often present in people with intellectual disabilities and autism spectrum disorder, who are diagnosed with schizophrenia (Bakken et al., 2008; O'Dwyer, 2000). A study comparing psychosis in people with intellectual disabilities, to those in the general population, found that negative symptoms were significantly more prevalent in the intellectual disabilities group. A Norwegian study reported that 26 participants with intellectual disabilities and autism spectrum disorder, diagnosed with psychosis, exhibited the following negative symptoms: fatigue, reduced initiative, and decreased social interaction (Bakken et al., 2023).

Observable Symptoms

Observable symptoms, especially aggression and self-mutilation, have been associated with mental health conditions in people with intellectual disabilities (Hausman et al., 2020; Painter et al., 2018). However, there is a complex relationship between such behaviours, and mental health conditions, as people with mental health conditions may or may not show dysfunctional regulation of emotions through actions. People with intellectual disabilities may exhibit behaviour that challenges for various reasons, including psychosis. Therefore, behavioural equivalents to symptoms of psychosis must be specifically attended to, beyond just observing challenging behaviour.

Behavioural equivalents should be observable symptoms corresponding to the criteria of psychosis as described in current assessment manuals. Using behavioural equivalents may increase the possibility of reaching a more accurate diagnosis, which can guide effective treatment and interventions (Bakken et al., 2007; Fletcher et al., 2016). Despite the advantages of using behavioural equivalents, it may decrease the validity of the diagnoses. Regarding psychosis, symptoms such as disorganized speech and behaviour (Bakken et al., 2007; Cherry et al., 2000) and negative symptoms (O'Dwyer, 2000) are directly observable. Delusions are not observable. Hallucinations may be interpreted through observations of possible hallucinatory behaviour (Bakken et al., 2007; Hurley, 2003). Behavioural equivalents should not be used as the sole source in the diagnostic process. Therefore, a multimodal assessment procedure is recommended (Bakken et al., 2023). An overview of observable symptoms is presented in the Table 2.1 (Bakken, 2021).

Conclusive Remarks

Psychotic symptoms can be observed in people with intellectual disabilities, ranging from mild to severe. Understanding the phenomenology for this group should include how symptoms vary at both the group and individual levels. The presentation of psychotic symptoms in people with intellectual disabilities is largely heterogeneous, due to the level of intellectual disabilities, additional neurodevelopmental conditions such as autism spectrum disorder, and individual idiosyncrasies. Knowledge about observable indicators of psychosis is helpful for both the assessment and treatment, especially during acute phases with high symptom

Table 2.1 Observable symptoms according to DSM-5 criteria (Bakken, 2021)

DSM-5 criteria		Observable symptoms
Criterion A Core symptoms	Delusions	Not observable when the person does not speak, or barely speaks
	Hallucinations	Hallucinatory behaviour including staring at fixed points and yelling, covering ears and at the same time uttering strange sounds, earaches without otitis, talks to himself out load, talks directly to people not there, talks out loud if upset, sensations not explainable, and says he sees things not there
	Disorganized speech	Incoherence/word salad, derailment, (severely) impoverished speech, speech vanished, meaningless response/ confused use of words (illogical speech), pressure of speech, and echolalia
	Disorganized behaviour	Derailment in task solving including task interruption by changing focus, sequence failure, aimlessness, rocking, repetitive behaviour, unexpected violent behaviour, meaningless response (non-verbal/gestures), using known objects wrongly (apraxia), impaired task solving in known activities
	Negative symptoms	Social withdrawal (more than usual, decreased number of initiatives), apathy/fatigue, lack of motivation (fewer initiatives than usual), blunted affect, lack of spontaneity
Criterion B Impaired functioning	Related to self-care, work, and relationships	Neglect related to self-care, work, and relationships. Tasks usually solved are neglected
Criterion C Duration	Continuous signs for at least 6 months	Not relevant regarding observable symptoms
	Criterion A symptoms for at least 1 month	Described above
Criterion D, E, F	Other conditions are ruled out	Not relevant regarding observable symptoms

load. Disorganized speech and behaviour, as well as negative symptoms, can be observed in people with mild, moderate, severe, and profound intellectual disabilities. Delusions cannot be observed directly but may be reported by people with mild and moderate intellectual disabilities. Hallucinations cannot be observed directly, but "hallucinatory behaviour" may be interpreted as hallucinations when observed concurrently with other psychotic symptoms.

References

Bakken, T. L. (2021). Behavioural equivalents of psychosis in people with intellectual disability and autism spectrum disorder. A selective review. *International Journal of Developmental Disabilities, 67*(5), 310–317.

Bakken, T. L., Eilertsen, D. E., Smeby, N. A., & Martinsen, H. (2008). Observing communication skills in staffs interacting with adults suffering from intellectual disability, autism and psychosis. *Nordic Journal of Nursing Research and Clinical Studies, 28*(1), 30–35.

Bakken, T. L., Eilertsen, D. E., Smeby, N. A., & Martinsen, H. (2009). The validity of disorganized behaviour as an indicator of psychosis in adults with autism and intellectual disability: A single case study. *Mental Health Aspects of Developmental Disabilities, 12*(1), 17–22.

Bakken, T. L., Friis, S., Løvoll, S., Smeby, N. A., & Martinsen, H. (2007). Behavioral disorganization as an indicator of psychosis in adults with intellectual disability and autism. *Mental Health Aspects of Developmental Disabilities, 10*(2), 37–46.

Bakken, T. L., & Høidal, S. H. (2014). Asperger syndrome or psychosis, or both? Case identification of 12 adults in a specialized psychiatric inpatient unit. *International Journal of Developmental Disabilities, 60*(4), 215–225.

Bakken, T. L., Kildahl, A. N., Ludvigsen, L. B., Bjørgen, T. G., Dalhaug, C., Hellerud, J. M. A., Hove, O., Solheim-Inderberg, A. M., Karlsen, K., & Helverschou, S. B. (2023). Psychosis in autistic people with intellectual disabilities: Symptom manifestations and identification. *Journal of Applied Research in Intellectual Disabilities.*

Baklund, L., Røssberg, J. I., Melbye, S. A., & Møller, P. (2024). Basic self-disturbance in adolescents at risk of psychosis: Temporal stability investigated by the experience sampling method in a mixed method study. *BMJ Ment Health, 27*(1).

Cherry, K. E., Penn, D., Matson, J. L., & Bamburg, J. W. (2000). Characteristics of psychosis among persons with severe or profound mental retardation. *Psychiatric Services, 51*(7), 922–924.

Engebretsen, M. H., Kildahl, A. N., Hoy, H. I., & Bakken, T. L. (2019). Metyrosine treatment in a woman with chromosome 22Q11.2 deletion syndrome and psychosis: A case study. *International Journal of Developemental Disabilities, 65*(2), 116–121.

Fletcher, R. J., Barnhill, J., & Cooper, S.-A. (2016). *Diagnostic manual—Intellectual disability. A textbook of diagnosis of mental disorders in persons with intellectual disability* (2nd ed.). DM-ID-2. The NADD Press.

Friedlander, R. I., & Donnelly, T. (2004). Early-onset psychosis in youth with intellectual disability. *Journal of Intellectual Disability Research, 48*(6), 540–547.

Hausman, N. L., Rooker, G. W., Bednar, M. K., & Javed, N. (2020). Considerations in the assessment and treatment of aggression and disruption. In J. Matson (Ed.), *Handbook of dual diagnosis. Autism and child psychopathology series.* Springer.

Heinimaa, M., Salokangas, R. K. R., Ristkari, T., Plathin, M., Huttunen, J., Ilonen, T., Suomela, T., Korkeila, J., & McGlashan, T. H. (2003). PROD-screen—A screen for prodromal symptoms of psychosis. *International Journal of Methods in Psychiatric Research, 12*(2), 92–104.

Hurley, A. D. (2003). Delusions and hallucinations in down syndrome: Literatures review and comparison with non-down-syndrome. *Mental Health Aspects of Developmental Disabilities, 6*, 135–146.

Noel, J. P., Cascio, C. J., Wallace, M. T., & Park, S. (2017). The spatial self in psychosis and autism spectrum disorder. *Psychosis Research, 179*, 8–12.

O'Dwyer, J. M. (2000). Autistic disorder and psychosis: Similarities and differences and their co-existence in two cases. *Mental Health Aspects of Developmental Disabilities, 3*, 121–131.

Painter, J., Hastings, R., Ingham, B., Trevithick, L., & Roy, A. (2018). Associations between mental health problems and challenging behavior in adults with intellectual disabilities: A test of the behavioral equivalents hypothesis. *Journal of Mental Health Research in Intellectual Disabilities, 11*(2), 157–172.

Parnas, J., Carter, J., & Nordgaard, J. (2016). Premorbid self-disorders and lifetime diagnosis in the schizophrenia spectrum: A prospective high-risk study. *Early Intervention in Psychiatry, 10*(1), 45–53.
Robinson, S., Howlin, P., & Russell, A. (2017). Personality traits, autobiographical memory and knowledge of self and others: A comparative study in young people with autism spectrum disorder. *Autism, 21*(3), 357–367.
Siegel, M., McGuire, K., Veenstra-VanderWeele, J., Stratigos, K., & King, B. (2020). American Academy of Child and Adolescent Psychiatry (AACAP) Committee on Quality Issues (CQI) practice parameter for the assessment and treatment of psychiatric disorders in children and adolescents with intellectual disability (intellectual developmental disorder). *Journal of the American Academy of Child and Adolescent Psychiatry, 59*, 468–496.
World Health Organization, WHO. (2018). ICD 11. *The 11th International Classification of Diseases*. WHO.

3

Diagnostic Assessment

Trine Lise Bakken

Abstract Diagnosis is a fundamental concept in medicine. A proper diagnosis is crucial, as it can lead to appropriate treatment and care. Two important areas in the diagnostic process for people with intellectual disabilities who are suspected of being psychotic are recognizing atypical symptoms and differentiating between challenging behaviour and psychotic symptoms. More about differential diagnostics will be covered in the next chapter. This chapter focuses on helpful tools in the diagnostic process, as well as the use of third-party information in addition to self-reports. The topics include clinical interviews, tools, and checklists: the Psychopathology in Autism Checklist (PAC), the Aberrant Behaviour Checklist (ABC), the MINI Plus Neuropsychiatric Interview, the Positive and Negative Syndrome Scale (PANSS), and the Diagnostic Manual—Intellectual Disability 2 (DM-ID 2).

T. L. Bakken (✉)
Oslo University Hospital, Oslo, Norway
e-mail: uxtlba@ous-hf.no

T. L. Bakken (ed.), *Psychosis in Adolescents and Adults with Intellectual Disabilities*,
https://doi.org/10.1007/978-3-031-95318-7_3

Keywords Atypical symptoms · Interdisciplinary team · Clinical interview · Diagnostic tools · Checklists · Self-report · Third-party information

The Diagnostic Process

The term "diagnosis" originates from Greek; "dia" and "gnosis," meaning "through knowledge." However, since mental health professionals use descriptive diagnoses not based on biological "proofs," the clinician and the team around the person should conduct the diagnostic work with humility and be aware of the risks of arriving at an unsuitable diagnosis.

Diagnostic assessment of psychosis in people with intellectual disabilities is complicated and resource-intensive (Bakken et al., 2023; Bertelli et al., 2015). The diagnostic work typically involves teamwork. The clinician in charge of the diagnostics needs to closely cooperate with a range of professionals and family members. The person in question should participate as much as possible, when not in the most acute phase. The assessment needs to be based on knowledge about intellectual disabilities, how intellectual disabilities impacts verbal functions at different levels, and knowledge about the phenomenology of psychotic symptoms and how they vary in the general population, and the population of people with intellectual disabilities. Clinical experience is important, and the lack of clinical experience may lead to misinterpretation of symptoms, and hence a wrong diagnosis (Bakken & Høidal, 2014). The large symptom overlaps between severe mental health conditions, especially psychosis, and cognitive impairments like intellectual disabilities and autism spectrum disorder may lead to misinterpretation of symptoms (Bertelli et al., 2015; Bradley et al., 2011).

Three factors particularly complicate the diagnostic assessment: similarity of symptoms between psychosis and autism spectrum disorder, or mental health/physical conditions, atypical symptoms, and the lack of ability to report on core psychotic symptoms (Bakken et al., 2023; Nylander, 2014). These factors may explain why symptoms of psychosis have previously been attributed to cognitive impairments themselves, and not an additional mental health condition, a phenomenon known as diagnostic overshadowing (Jopp & Keys, 2001).

The practical diagnostic work is usually conducted through a combination of clinical interviews and the use of diagnostic tools/checklists, combined with comparative information. In addition, case files may be useful. Such information may be obtained from the person's general practitioner, professional caregivers in community services, pedagogues and pedagogues at school for children and adolescents, other milieu therapists in community services, family members and/or acquaintances, as well as case files, if available. If the person, for various reasons, cannot report on potentially psychotic symptoms, the use of behavioural equivalents to conventional symptoms may be a feasible solution (see Chapter 2).

Diagnostic Tools and Checklists

There are a number of checklists available for screening mental health conditions in people with intellectual disabilities. For a more comprehensive presentation of both checklists and clinical interviews, see Helverschou et al. (2020).

The Psychopathology in Autism Checklist (PAC) (Bakken et al., 2010; Helverschou et al., 2009) encompasses five subscales and 42 items: general adjustment problems (GAP) 12 items, psychosis 10 items, depression 7 items, anxiety 6 items, and OCD 7 items. Each item is rated in two domains: extent of problems (1–4) and change in usual behaviour (worsened, unchanged, improved). A two-step procedure identifies people with a possible mental health condition. First, people with severe general adjustment problems are identified (GAP score > cut-off). Individuals who also obtain a score above the cut-off for any of the four specific scales are classified as having a suspected mental health condition. In a study of a clinical sample of 26 adults with intellectual disabilities and autism spectrum disorder assessed for psychosis (Bakken et al., 2023), the PAC showed overall good internal consistency (Cronbach's $\alpha = 0.90$), as well as for PAC psychosis ($\alpha = 0.77$).

The Aberrant Behavior Checklist (ABC) (Aman & Sing, 1986) was developed to measure challenging behaviour. As psychotic conditions may include anxiety and hence aggression, the ABC may be feasible for measuring treatment effects (Bakken et al., 2024). The use of the

ABC is widespread for the assessment of challenging behaviour (Helverschou et al., 2020; Aman & Sing, 1986). The psychometric properties have been found to vary from satisfactory to excellent (Flynn et al., 2017; Helverschou et al., 2020). The ABC encompasses 58 items constituting five subscales: irritability 15 items, lethargy 16 items, stereotypic behaviour 7 items, hyperactivity 16 items, and inappropriate speech 4 items. Items are rated using a four-point scale (not a problem—severe problem). In the same sample mentioned for the PAC, the overall internal consistency of the ABC was good (Cronbach's $\alpha = 0.94$).

The MINI Plus neuropsychiatric interview (Sheehan et al., 1998) may be feasible when the person is not in the most acute phase. Within the general population, it is recommended to score all modules in the MINI Plus. It is estimated that the MINI Plus can be scored in less than an hour. However, this may not be possible for persons with intellectual disabilities and additional psychosis. Bakken and Høidal (2014) used relevant modules from the MINI Plus based on the scores from the PAC, combined with the reasons for referral in 12 persons with intellectual disabilities diagnosed with or suspected of having psychosis. The participants were scored for the modules A (major depression), D (mania), E (panic disorder), and M (psychosis). Scoring as many modules as possible from the MINI Plus may be helpful for differential diagnostic purposes. The MINI Plus may also be a helpful tool when conducting a clinical interview.

The Positive and Negative Syndrome Scale (PANSS) (Kay et al., 1987) is a widely used tool for the assessment of symptoms in persons with psychosis (Opler et al., 2017). It is used for measuring symptom severity of psychosis and is widely used in medication studies. The scale is a 30-item clinician-administered rating scale. It is estimated to take about an hour. However, the interviewer needs training due to the complexity of the scale (Peralta & Cuesta, 1994). The PANSS requires 45–50 minutes to be administered by a trained clinician. The PANSS is mostly used for grading symptom severity in psychosis. It quantifies positive and negative symptoms. The PANSS encompasses three subscales: positive scale, negative scale, and general psychopathology scale (Kay et al., 1987). The PANSS has adequate internal consistency, good test–retest reliability, and inter-rater reliability (Peralta & Cuesta, 1994). The PANSS has been investigated and found to be promising also for persons with mild intellectual disabilities (Hatton et al., 2005).

The last tool in this chapter is the DM-ID 2, Diagnostic Manual—Intellectual Disability 2 (Fletcher et al., 2016). The DM-ID 2 is a comprehensive diagnostic manual, including a "state of the art" section, descriptions of symptoms, and a reference list for each chapter. The DM-ID 2 is based on the DSM-5, published in 2013 (American Psychiatric Association), and reflects the changes from DSM-4 to DSM-5 (Fletcher et al., 2016). The DM-ID 2 chapter on schizophrenia and other psychoses includes a review of research literature, diagnostic criteria, and an introduction on how to apply diagnostic criteria to people with intellectual disabilities. It then presents the different diagnostic categories with criteria and descriptions on application for mild/moderate intellectual disabilities and severe/profound intellectual disabilities, respectively. The DM-ID is thorough, and the specific descriptions on applications for mild/moderate and severe/profound intellectual disabilities may be helpful for clinicians conducting the assessment. The DM-ID may also be helpful as a guide for professional caregivers, especially intellectual disabilities nurses and mental health nurses when observing possible psychotic symptoms.

Clinical Interview

As mentioned above, impairments of language and introspection will worsen in people with intellectual disabilities when they develop psychotic conditions. Clinical interviews may not be possible to carry out during acute or sub-acute phases when the person shows fragmented thinking (disorganization) and language issues (Bakken et al., 2009). However, if the diagnosis on the psychosis spectrum is reached by gathering data from multiple sources, a clinical interview may be feasible to validate the diagnosis when the person is in remission (Engebretsen et al., 2019). The clinician should be aware of pitfalls when the person has intellectual disabilities. Two aspects are especially important: "yes-saying" and impaired ability of abstraction. "Yes-saying" is a well-known phenomenon among researchers. The concept refers to the informant wanting to agree or make a positive impression (Finlay & Lyons, 2001; Sauro & Lewis, 2011). The ability of abstraction may also be a challenge. A study at Oslo University Hospital on ward atmosphere (emotional climate) showed that persons with intellectual disabilities and additional severe mental conditions (psychosis, bipolar disorders, or major depression) had significant problems with answering a four-point scale on ward atmosphere (Sommerstad et al., 2021). Instead of the mentioned scale, a design with open-ended questions was used (Sommerstad et al., 2021). Generally, the use of abstractions like "usually" should be avoided in clinical interviews. It is usually better to ask if something occurs every day, multiple times a day, or weekly (Finlay & Lyons, 2001). Also "often" or "very often" are examples of difficult concepts.

An advantage of using the MINI Plus when assessing people with intellectual disabilities is the thorough descriptions of the symptoms. Each symptom presentation may be read to the person, who can then confirm or deny the symptom being present. Persons with intellectual disabilities who are suspected of suffering from psychosis may have considerable problems reporting symptoms, even when they are not in the most acute phase. Hence, the descriptions in the MINI Plus may be difficult to recognize, or the person may not be used to reporting signs of mental ill-health (Bakken et al., 2023). A solution to this problem may be training with the person. For example, "Carl" was in his thirties and had visited a number of clinicians without being provided any diagnosis or explanation of his difficult life. At the time of assessment using the MINI Plus with a trained clinician, he was staying in reinforced housing with 3:1 staffing around the clock. The clinician visited twice a week. Instead of starting with the MINI Plus immediately, Carl practised answering general questions repeatedly. His regular way of answering was to state "not right" or "right." For example, the response to "Carl is a woman" would be "not right." The difficulty level of the training increased until Carl was able to evaluate the content of the symptom descriptions in the MINI Plus.

Person Reported Symptoms

As people with intellectual disabilities and additional psychotic conditions usually are severely disturbed during acute phases, a diagnosis of psychosis should not be validated until the person is in remission and verbal abilities are regained (Engebretsen et al., 2019). People with intellectual disabilities may have problems reporting inner experiences, even if they can express themselves in their everyday life. Moreover, professional caregivers may be more concerned about challenging behaviour than people with intellectual disabilities themselves (Rose et al., 2013). In a study on anger and intellectual disabilities, participants with mild and moderate intellectual disabilities reported having more internal emotions and mental health problems, whereas professional caregivers reported more challenging behaviour (Rose et al., 2013).

More research addresses this discrepancy between person-reported symptoms and family/professional caregiver-reported symptoms (Douma et al., 2006; Finlay & Lyons, 2001; Moss et al., 1996; Scott & Havercamp, 2018). Generally, person-reported outcome measures (PROM) have been found to be more clinically relevant for interventions than measures reported by clinicians alone (Mercieca-Bebber et al., 2017). Already in 1996, Moss and colleagues reported that adults with mild and moderate intellectual disabilities reported more anxiety and depression than community caregivers reported. The latter group reported more stress and psychotic symptoms.

Conclusive Remarks

Most of the tools presented in this chapter use professional caregiver reports or family member reports. However, studies indicate that individuals with intellectual disabilities report more mental health problems, whereas caregivers report more behavioural problems. This discrepancy should encourage clinicians to use third-party information with caution and seek information from multiple sources.

References

Aman, M. G., & Sing, N. N. (1986). *Aberrant behavior checklist*. Slossen Educational.

Bakken, T. L., Askeland Hellerud, J. M., Kildahl, A. N., Solheim-Inderberg, A. M., Berge Helverschou, S., & Hove, O. (2024). Psychosis in autistic people with intellectual disabilities. Treatment and interventions. *Journal of Autism and Developmental Disorders,* 1–11.

Bakken, T. L., Eilertsen, D. E., Smeby, N. A., & Martinsen, H. (2009). The validity of disorganised behaviour as an indicator of psychosis in adults with autism and intellectual disability: A single case study. *Mental Health Aspects of Developmental Disabilities, 12*(1), 17–22.

Bakken, T. L., Helverschou, S. B., Eilertsen, D. E., Hegglund, T., Myrbakk, E., & Martinsen, H. (2010). Psychiatric disorders in adolescents and adults with autism and intellectual disability: A representative study in one county in Norway. *Research in Developmental Disabilities, 31*(6), 1669–1677.

Bakken, T. L., & Høidal, S. H. (2014). Asperger syndrome or psychosis, or both? Case identification of 12 adults in a specialised psychiatric inpatient unit. *International Journal of Developmental Disabilities, 60*(4), 215–225.

Bakken, T. L., Kildahl, A. N., Ludvigsen, L. B., Bjørgen, T. G., Dalhaug, C., Hellerud, J. M. A., Hove, O., Solheim-Inderberg, A. M., Karlsen, K., & Helverschou, S. B. (2023). Psychosis in autistic people with intellectual disabilities: Symptom manifestations and identification. *Journal of Applied Research in Intellectual Disabilities.*

Bertelli, M. O., Piva Merli, M., Bradley, E., Keller, R., Varrucciu, N., Del Furia, C., & Panocchia, N. (2015). The diagnostic boundary between autism spectrum disorder, intellectual developmental disorder and schizophrenia spectrum disorders. *Advances in Mental Health and Intellectual Disabilities, 9*(5), 243–264.

Bradley, E., Lunsky, Y., Palucka, A., & Homitidis, S. (2011). Recognition of intellectual disabilities and autism in psychiatric inpatients diagnosed with schizophrenia and other psychotic disorders. *Advances in Mental Health and Intellectual Disabilities, 5*(6), 4–18.

Douma, J. C. H., Dekker, M. C., Verhulst, F. C., & Koot, H. M. (2006). Self-reports on mental health problems of youth with moderate to borderline intellectual disabilities. *Journal of American Child & Adolescent Psychiatry, 45*(10), 1224–1231.

Engebretsen, M. H., Kildahl, A. N., Høy, H. I., & Bakken, T. L. (2019). Metyrosine treatment in a woman with chromosome 22Q11.2 deletion syndrome and psychosis: A case study. *International Journal of Developmental Disabilities, 65*(2), 116–121.

Finlay, W. M., & Lyons, E. (2001). Methodological issues in interviewing and using self-report questionnaires with people with mental retardation. *Psychological Assessment, 13*(3), 319.

Fletcher, R. J., Barnhill, J., & Cooper, S.-A. (2016). *Diagnostic manual—Intellectual disability: A textbook of diagnosis of mental disorders in persons with intellectual disability, DM-ID 2.* NADD Press.

Fletcher, R. J., Barnhill, J., McCarthy, J., & Strydom, A. (2016). From DSM to DM-ID. *Journal of Mental Health Research in Intellectual Disabilities, 9*(3), 189–204.

Flynn, S., Vereenooghe, L., Hastings, R. P., Adams, D., Cooper, S. A., Gore, N., Hatton, C., Hood, K., Jahoda, A., Langdon, P. E., McNamara, R., Oliver, C., Roy, A., Totsika, V., & Waite, J. (2017). Measurement tools for mental health problems and mental well-being in people with severe or profound intellectual disabilities: A systematic review. *Clinical Psychology Review, 57*, 32–44.

Hatton, C., Haddock, G., Taylor, J. L., Coldwell, J., Crossley, R., & Peckham, N. (2005). The reliability and validity of general psychotic rating scales with people with mild and moderate intellectual disabilities: An empirical investigation. *Journal of Intellectual Disability Research, 49*(7), 490–500.

Helverschou, S. B., Bakken, T. L., & Martinsen, H. (2009). The psychopathology in autism checklist (PAC): A pilot study. *Research in Autism Spectrum Disorders, 3*(1), 179–195.

Helverschou, S. B., Kildahl, A. N., & Bakken, T. L. (2020). Checklists and structured interviews. In J. L. Matson (Ed.), *Handbook of dual diagnosis*, Autism and child psychopathology series.

Jopp, D. A., & Keys, C. B. (2001). Diagnostic overshadowing reviewed and reconsidered. *American Journal on Mental Retardation, 106*(5), 416–433.

Kay, S. R., Fiszbein, A., & Opler, L. A. (1987). The positive and negative syndrome scale (PANSS) for psychosis. *Schizophrenia Bulletin, 13*(2), 261–276.

Mercieca-Bebber, R., Firedlander, M., calvert, M., Stockler, M., Kyte, D., Kok, P. S., & King, M. T. (2017). A systematic evaluation of compliance and reporting of person-reported outcome endpoints in ovarian cancer randomised controlled trials: Implications for generalisability and clinical practice. *Journal of Person-reported Outcomes, 1*(5), 2457–2465.

Moss, S., Prosser, H., Ibbotson, B., & Goldberg, D. (1996). Respondent and informant accounts of psychiatric symptoms in a sample of patients with learning disability. *Journal of Intellectual Disability Research, 40*(5), 457–465.

Nylander, L. (2014). Autism and psychosis in adults: Clinical considerations on comorbidity and differential diagnosis. In V. B. Patel, V. R. Preedy, & C. R. Martin (Eds.), *Comprehensive guide to autism* (pp. 585–600). Springer.

Opler, M. G., Yavorsky, C., & Daniel, D. G. (2017). Positive and negative syndrome scale (PANSS) training: Challenges, solutions, and future directions. *Innovations in Clinical Neuroscience, 14*(11–12), 77.

Peralta, V., & Cuesta, M. J. (1994). Psychometric properties of the positive and negative syndrome scale (PANSS) in schizophrenia. *Psychiatry Research, 53*(1), 31–40.

Rose, J., Willner, P., Shead, J., Jahoda, A., Gillespie, D., Townson, J., Lammie, C., Woodgate, C., Kroese, B. S., Felce, D., MacMahon, P., Rose, N., Stimpson, A., Nuttall, J., & Hood, K. (2013). Different factors influence self-reports and third-party reports of anger by adults with intellectual disabilities. *Journal of Applied Research in Intellectual Disabilities, 26*(5), 410–419.

Sauro, J., & Lewis, J. R. (2011 May). When designing usability questionnaires, does it hurt to be positive? In *Proceedings of the SIGCHI conference on human factors in computing systems* (pp. 2215–2224).

Scott, H. M., & Havercamp, S. M. (2018). Comparisons of self and proxy report on health-related factors in people with intellectual disability. *Journal of Applied Research in Intellectual Disabilities, 31*(5), 927–936.

Sheehan, D. V., Lecrubier, Y., Sheehan, K. H., Amorim, P., Janavs, J., Weiller, E., Hergueta, T., Baker, R., & Dunbar, G. C. (1998). The mini-international neuropsychiatric interview (MINI): The development and validation of a structured diagnostic psychiatric interview for DSM-IV and ICD-10. *Journal of Clinical Psychiatry, 59*(20), 22–33.

Sommerstad, H. S., Kildahl, A. N., Munkhaugen, E. K., Karlsen, K., & Bakken, T. L. (2021). Experiences of ward atmosphere in inpatients with intellectual disability and mental illness. Clinical implications for mental health nursing. *International Journal of Developmental Disabilities, 67*(5), 339–348.

4
Differential Diagnostics

Trine Lise Bakken

Abstract The differential diagnostic assessment, including the exclusion of other explanations for the symptoms, encompasses a number of factors that may complicate the diagnostic assessment of psychosis in people with intellectual disabilities. Several conditions may be mistaken for psychosis in people with intellectual disabilities. In this chapter, the following areas are addressed as possible differential diagnostic categories to psychosis: autism spectrum disorder, obsessive–compulsive disorder (OCD), post-traumatic stress disorder (PTSD), neurological disorders, and physical disorders causing pain.

Keywords Differential diagnosis · Autism spectrum disorder · Obsessive–compulsive disorder · Post-traumatic stress disorder · Neurological disorder · Physical pain

T. L. Bakken (✉)
Oslo University Hospital, Oslo, Norway
e-mail: uxtlba@ous-hf.no

T. L. Bakken (ed.), *Psychosis in Adolescents and Adults with Intellectual Disabilities*,
https://doi.org/10.1007/978-3-031-95318-7_4

Diagnostic Obstacles

As mental health diagnoses are still descriptive in nature, the clinician has to base the diagnosis on two information sources: what the person reports and what can be observed. As mentioned in Chapter 3, language and introspection impairments will worsen in people with intellectual disabilities when they develop psychotic conditions. This leaves the clinician predominantly with observations, noting the decline in the person's ability to maintain self-care, relationships, and adaptive functioning. Diagnostic overshadowing, overlapping symptoms, and atypical symptom presentation mainly complicate the identification of psychosis in adolescents and adults with intellectual disabilities. Diagnostic overshadowing is a phenomenon where symptoms of mental health conditions are attributed to the person's intellectual disabilities rather than a mental health condition (Jopp & Keys, 2001; Reiss et al., 1982). The same phenomenon occurs in relation to autism spectrum disorder. When behaviour changes, deterioration of language, or emotional dysregulation are attributed to intellectual disabilities, psychosis may be overlooked. People with all levels of intellectual disabilities may appear agitated and exhibit signs of psychological stress in different situations, not only when experiencing a psychotic disorder. A special kind of diagnostic overshadowing is the phenomenon where the person's behaviour is explained as characteristics of their personality instead of a mental health condition (Wadel, 1990). Terms like "idleness," "activity denial," "wanting attention," "escaping from tasks," or "trying to trick the staff" are commonly used explanations in clinical practice.

Overlapping symptoms occur especially in people at all levels of intellectual disabilities. Persons who are not able to express their inner feelings tend to express themselves through actions. For example, negative symptoms resemble features of autism. Likewise, hearing voices is usually stressful for the person, who may scream or throw items (Bakken et al., 2007), which resembles features of anxiety or may be defined as behaviour that challenges. Atypical symptoms also appear more often in people with more severe intellectual disabilities (Ghaziuddin, 2005). Impaired language skills are closely related to the occurrence of behaviour that challenges, and stereotyped activity. Repetitive behaviour and behaviour that challenges behaviour that challenges (violence, damaging objects, or self-mutilation) have been identified as atypical symptoms of mental health issues in persons with both intellectual disabilities and autism spectrum disorders (Myers & Winters, 2002; Tantam, 2000).

Autism Spectrum Disorder or Psychosis?

There are a number of symptoms that may be attributed to both autism and psychosis, especially delusions, thought disorder, and negative symptoms (Bakken & Hoidal, 2014; Bakken et al., 2007, 2023; Nylander, 2014). Additionally, high levels of stress may be observed in both diagnostic groups (Bakken et al., 2007; Nylander, 2014).

Idiosyncratic language and opinions, and a personal way of behaving in people with autism may be mistaken for delusions. Features of thought disorder (manifested by disorganized speech) are found in both people with psychosis and autism (Konstantareas & Hewitt, 2001; Rumsey et al., 1986). However, people with autism tend to show more features of disorganized speech, observed as impoverished language, deviant responses, and inappropriate thinking (Konstantareas & Hewitt, 2001; Rumsey et al., 1986). Features of disorganized speech are one of the core symptom groups of psychosis (Andreasen, 1979). People with psychosis will tend to show more incoherent speech, pressure of speech, and derailment than people with autism (Konstantareas & Hewitt, 2001; Rumsey et al., 1986). Symptoms may be wrongly attributed during the diagnostic assessment when one relies on thought disorder as characteristic feature of psychosis without ruling out autism. In a study from 2014 (Bakken & Hoidal, 2014), two persons in a convenient sample study showed grossly disorganized speech, consistent with psychosis. The two persons showed incoherence, pressure of speech, derailment, and impoverished speech. Their disorganized behaviour and speech had previously been attributed to autism. People with autism have cognitive and information-processing impairments, which affect their thinking and language (Volkmar et al., 2004), which must be taken into consideration when a diagnosis on the psychosis spectrum is suspected.

Regarding negative symptoms, research has found large areas of overlap between autism and psychosis (Bakken & Hoidal, 2014; Bakken et al., 2007). Low social activity, lack of motivation, and affect flattening can be attributed to both autism and psychosis (Konstantareas & Hewitt, 2001; Rumsey et al., 1986). Negative symptoms in psychosis, especially apathy, may remain over longer periods when the person is in remission and are the core symptoms of psychosis that are hard to treat with antipsychotic medication (Faerden et al., 2010). Long-lasting negative symptoms have the potential to be confused with social withdrawal in autism. In the Bakken and Hoidal study (2014), 3 persons out of 12 showed severe negative symptoms that had previously been misinterpreted as core features of autism.

In people with more severe intellectual disabilities, the risk of misinterpretation of symptoms will likely occur more often than in those with mild or moderate intellectual disabilities, who may report core symptoms when they are in remission.

Obsessive–Compulsive Disorder or Psychosis?

The overlap between obsessive–compulsive disorder (OCD) and psychosis in the general population is considerable (Mawn et al., 2020; Tonna et al., 2016). An Italian clinical study included about 60 people with either psychosis or OCD, with approximately 30 in each group (Tonna et al., 2016). Symptoms were obtained by self-report and interviews using the Yale-Brown Obsessive Compulsive Scale (Y-BOCS) (Goodman et al., 1989). The two groups did not differ significantly in the total Y-BOCS symptom scores regarding both obsessions and compulsions. Additionally, there were no differences in symptom activity at the group level. However, a closer look at the phenomenology revealed differences. The OCD group showed higher levels of stress related to both obsessions and compulsions, and more aggressive, contamination-related, sexual, and somatic obsessions compared to the psychosis group. The psychosis group showed more washing and hoarding behaviours. Similar results are found in people with intellectual disabilities (Dalhaug et al., 2023). However, symptoms of OCD may be easily observed through behaviours such as counting or obsessive cleaning, while psychotic symptoms mainly manifest as inner, subjective experiences. There seems to be a risk that psychotic symptoms may be overlooked in persons with intellectual disabilities showing OCD symptomatology (Dalhaug et al., 2023). Obsessions in OCD and delusions in psychosis may be challenging to distinguish at a phenomenological level, particularly in people with intellectual disabilities. Mawn and colleagues (2020) recommend that people diagnosed with psychosis should be examined for OCD, and vice versa. The results of Dalhaug and colleagues (2023) suggest that the same procedure should be applied to people with intellectual disabilities.

Post-traumatic Stress Disorder or Psychosis?

People with intellectual disabilities seem to be more vulnerable to intrusive behaviour and experiencing potentially traumatic events (Kildahl et al., 2020; Mevissen et al., 2016), and may hence be at higher risk for developing post-traumatic stress disorder (PTSD). PTSD symptoms may be difficult to distinguish from both anxiety and psychosis, leading to frequent misinterpretation of such symptoms (Kildahl et al., 2020; Mevissen et al., 2016). Intrusive memories or flashbacks, in particular, may be misinterpreted as hallucinations or delusions if family members or professional caregivers are unaware of the traumatic experience and therefore unable to interpret the person's behaviour in light of this experience. Obtaining a trauma history during assessment may be helpful (Kildahl & Jørstad, 2022).

A clinical study presented the assessment of possible trauma in five adults with intellectual disabilities in a specialized mental health inpatient unit (Bakken et al., 2014). Three of the participants were previously medicated for psychotic illness due to severe psychopathology, such as a severe decline in self-care and task-solving, high levels of psychological stress, and anxiety attacks. However, new assessments using the Lancaster and Northgate Trauma Scales (LANTS Scale) (Wigham et al., 2011), revealed trauma symptoms in the five participants. Four of the participants had experienced sexual abuse and the loss of family members.

The fifth participant had spent her childhood in a central institution, where she had repeatedly been secluded and strapped to her bed. One of the participant's retellings of the story about sexual abuse had previously been considered inappropriate and interpreted as psychotic delusions.

Neurological Disorders, Pain or Psychosis?

Neurological disorders may be difficult to separate from psychosis, as the two often occur in the same person (Danielyan & Nasrallah, 2009). Some frequently occurring neurological disorders, especially epilepsy, which causes seizures and brain dysfunction, may cause hallucinations, illusions, and/or delusions (Kasper et al., 2010). These symptoms may appear not only during seizures or post-seizure, but at any conscious moment (Danielyan & Nasrallah, 2009). As people with intellectual disabilities significantly more often suffer from both psychotic illness and neurological disorders, both groups of disorders should be considered in the assessment.

People diagnosed with psychotic conditions significantly more often experience physical conditions compared to the general population (Kugathasan et al., 2019). This is also the case for people with intellectual disabilities (Glover et al., 2017). Hence, professionals in mental health services, who have the responsibility for their care, should be particularly vigilant in monitoring and addressing physical health issues in these populations.

People diagnosed with psychotic conditions significantly more often experience physical illnesses compared to the general population (Kugathasan et al., 2019). This is also the case for people with intellectual disabilities (Glover et al., 2017). Hence, professionals in mental health services, who have the responsibility for their care, should be particularly vigilant in monitoring and addressing physical health issues in these populations.

Physical pain can also be confused with psychosis. People with intellectual disabilities may show pain, especially severe pain, in unusual ways, such as agitation, aggression towards others, self-mutilation, and/or shouting (Sappok et al., 2019). These behaviours can also be observed in acute phases of psychosis in people with intellectual disabilities (Bakken et al., 2007). Psychotic disorganized behaviour could be mistaken for challenging behaviour, which resembles the behaviours described by Sappok and colleagues (2019). Hence, physical pain should be considered in people with intellectual disabilities suspected of having psychosis.

Conclusive Remarks

Psychosis may be hard to detect in people with intellectual disabilities. Therefore, both mental health and physical conditions should be considered when psychosis is suspected in people with intellectual disabilities. A thorough physical examination should be conducted, including blood tests and screening for toothache and other conditions that typically cause physical pain. Additionally, since co-morbid mental health conditions are common in people with schizophrenia, a comprehensive mental health screening should be provided.

References

Andreasen, N. C. (1979). Thought, language, and communication disorders. *Archives of General Psychiatry, 36*, 1315–1321.

Bakken, T. L., Friis, S., Lovoll, S., Smeby, N. A., & Martinsen, H. (2007). Behavioral disorganisation as an indicator of psychosis in adults with intellectual disability and autism. *Mental Health Aspects of Developmental Disabilities, 10*(2), 37–46.

Bakken, T. L., & Hoidal, S. H. (2014). Asperger syndrome or psychosis, or both? Case identification of 12 adults in a specialised psychiatric inpatient unit. *International Journal of Developmental Disabilities, 60*(4), 215–225.

Bakken, T. L., Kildahl, A. N., Gjersøe, V., Matre, E., Kristiansen, T., Ro, A., Tveter A. L., & Hoidal, S. H. (2014). Identification of PTSD in adults with intellectual disabilities in five patients in a specialised psychiatric inpatient unit. *Advances in Mental Health and Intellectual Disabilities, 8*(2), 91–102.

Bakken, T. L., Kildahl, A. N., Ludvigsen, L. B., Bjørgen, T. G., Dalhaug, C., Hellerud, J. M. A., Hove, O., Solheim-Inderberg, A. M., Karlsen, K., &

Helverschou, S. B. (2023). Psychosis in autistic people with intellectual disabilities: Symptom manifestations and identification. *Journal of Applied Research in Intellectual Disabilities.*

Dalhaug, K. C., Storvik, K., & Kildahl, A. N. (2023). Undiagnosed psychotic disorder in autistic persons with intellectual disabilities and suspected obsessive-compulsive disorder: An explorative, clinical study. *Journal of Mental Health Research in Intellectual Disabilities, 16*(3), 226–252.

Danielyan, A., & Nasrallah, H. A. (2009). Neurological disorders in psychosis. *Psychiatric Clinics, 32*(4), 719–757.

Faerden, A., Finset, A., Friis, S., Agartz, I., Barrett, E. A., Nesvåg, R., Andreassen, O. A., Marder, S. R., & Melle, I. (2010). Apathy in first episode psychosis patients: One year follow up. *Psychosis Research, 116*(1), 20–26.

Ghaziuddin, M. (2005). *Mental health aspects of autism and Asperger syndrome.* Jessica Kingsley Publishers.

Glover, G., Williams, R., Heslop, P., Oyinlola, J., & Grey, J. (2017). Mortality in people with intellectual disabilities in England. *Journal of Intellectual Disability Research, 61*(1), 62–74.

Goodman, W. K., Price, L. H., Rasmussen, S. A., et al. (1989). The Yale-Brown obsessive compulsive scale. I. Development, use, and reliability. *Archives of General Psychiatry, 46*, 1006–1011.

Jopp, D. A., & Keys, C. B. (2001). Diagnostic overshadowing reviewed and reconsidered. *American Journal on Mental Retardation, 106*(5), 416–433.

Kasper, B. S., Taylor, D. C., Janz, D., Kasper, E. M., Maier, M., Williams, M. R., & Crow, T. J. (2010). Neuropathology of epilepsy and psychosis: The contributions of JAN Corsellis. *Brain, 133*(12), 3795–3805.

Kildahl, A. N., Helverschou, S. B., Bakken, T. L., & Oddli, H. W. (2020). "If we do not look for it, we do not see it"; Clinicians experiences and understanding of identifying post-traumatic stress disorder in adults autism and intellectual disability. *Journal of Research in Intellectual Disabilities, 00*, 1–14.

Kildahl, A. N., & Jørstad, I. (2022). Post-traumatic stress disorder symptom manifestations in an autistic man with severe intellectual disability following coercion and scalding. *Journal of Intellectual & Developmental Disability, 47*(2), 190–194.

Konstantareas, M. M., & Hewitt, T. (2001). Autistic disorder and psychosis: Diagnostic overlaps. *Journal of Autism and Developmental Disorders, 31*(1), 19–28.

Kugathasan, P., Stubbs, B., Aagaard, J., Jensen, S. E., Munk Laursen, T., & Nielsen, R. E. (2019). Increased mortality from somatic multimorbidity in patients with schizophrenia: A Danish nationwide cohort study. *Acta Psychiatrica Scandinavica, 140*(4), 340–348.

Mawn, L., Campbell, T., Aynsworth, C., Beckwith, H., Luce, A., Barclay, N., Dodgson, G., & Freeston, M. H. (2020). Comorbidity of obsessive-compulsive and psychotic experiences: A systematic review and meta-analysis. *Journal of Obsessive-Compulsive and Related Disorders, 26*, 100539.

Mevissen, L., Didden, R., & de Jongh, A. (2016). Assessment and treatment of PTSD in people with intellectual disabilities. In *Comprehensive guide to post-traumatic stress disorder* (pp. 281–299).

Myers, K., & Winters, N. C. (2002). Ten-year review of rating scales, II: Scales for internalising disorders. *The Journal of the American Academy of Child & Adolescent Psychiatry's, 41*, 634–659.

Nylander, L. (2014). Autism and psychosis in adults: Clinical considerations on comorbidity and differential diagnosis. In V. B. Patel, V. R. Preedy, & C. R. Martin (Eds.), *Comprehensive guide to autism* (pp. 585–600). Springer.

Reiss, S., Levitan, G. W., & Szyszko, J. (1982). Emotional disturbance and mental retardation: Diagnostic overshadowing. *American Journal of Mental Deficiency, 86*(6), 567–574.

Rumsey, J. M., Andreasen, N. C., & Rapoport, J. L. (1986). Thought, language, communication and affective flattening in autistic adults. *Archives of General Psychiatry, 43*, 771–777.

Sappok, T., Diefenbacher, A., & Winterholler, M. (2019). The medical care of people with intellectual disability. *Deutsches Ärzteblatt International, 116*(48), 809.

Tantam, D. (2000). Psychological disorder in adolescents and adults with Asperger syndrome. *Autism, 4*(1), 47–62.

Tonna, M., Ottoni, R., Paglia, F., Monici, A., Ossola, P., De Panfilis, C., & Marchesi, C. (2016). Obsessive-compulsive symptoms in psychosis and in obsessive-compulsive disorder: Differences and similarities. *Journal of Psychiatric Practice, 22*(2), 111–116.

Volkmar, F. R., Lord, C., Bailey, A., Schultz, R. T., & Klin, A. (2004). Autism and pervasive developmental disorders. *Journal of Child Psychology and Psychiatry, 45*(1), 135–170.

Wadel, C. (1990). *The social scientific construction of reality* [Den samfunnsvitenskapelige konstruksjon av virkeligheten], SEEK.

Wigham, S., Hatton, C., & Taylor, J. L. (2011). The Lancaster and Northgate Trauma Scales (LANTS): The development and psychometric properties of a measure of trauma for people with mild to moderate intellectual disabilities. *Research in Developmental Disabilities, 32*(6), 2651–2659.

5

Adaptive Skills and Emotional Development

Kjersti Karlsen

Abstract Both intellectual disabilities and psychosis are complex conditions affecting cognitive, adaptive, and emotional functioning. Moreover, psychosis is associated with lower cognitive functioning compared to the general population, particularly in those with early onset or very early onset. Adaptive skills are intertwined with cognitive abilities. For persons with both intellectual disabilities and psychosis, adaptive skills may be severely impaired during high-symptom phases. Impairments of emotional development is not one of the main criteria of intellectual disabilities. However, emotional development is delayed and impaired in this group. This chapter describes why emotional development is an important area of knowledge. Emotional development is strongly related to behavioural expressions. Hence, understanding the level of emotional development is crucial for understanding challenging behaviour in people with intellectual disabilities who develop psychosis. A tool for assessing emotional development will be presented.

K. Karlsen (✉)
Oslo University Hospital, Oslo, Norway
e-mail: uxkkje@ous-hf.no

T. L. Bakken (ed.), *Psychosis in Adolescents and Adults with Intellectual Disabilities*,
https://doi.org/10.1007/978-3-031-95318-7_5

Keywords Cognition · Adaptive skills · Emotional development · The SEED-2

Cognition in Intellectual Disabilities

IQ is directly linked to intellectual disabilities, as one of the two main criteria for diagnosis is an IQ below 70. However, this can deviate if the IQ is slightly higher than 70 and adaptive skills are significantly impaired. People with intellectual disabilities generally have low cognitive abilities across various cognitive domains. Although the cognitive profile may be uneven, it shows a stable pattern since childhood (American Psychiatric Association, APA, 2013). Sudden changes in thinking, perception, or behaviour are not consistent with a diagnosis of intellectual disabilities. Core cognitive domains include executive functions (including working memory), attention and concentration, memory, language and verbal functions, visual/visuospatial functions, and social cognition.

Cognition in Psychosis

Psychosis is associated with cognitive deficits, and professionals may prefer to classify it as a neurodevelopmental disorder (Smelror & Ueland, 2023). The most affected cognitive domains include executive functions, verbal fluency, attention, and processing speed (Zhang et al., 2024). The type and degree of cognitive impairments depend on both the age of onset and symptom variation in psychosis, leading to significant variability among individuals diagnosed with psychosis. Cognitive decline may be inherent or begin months to years before the onset of psychosis. It can also be a direct consequence of psychotic symptoms, fluctuating with symptom severity, though it often occurs independently of psychosis. Furthermore, cognitive decline is generally observed to occur independently of medication (Zhang et al., 2024).

Adolescent and adult onset of psychosis is associated with cognitive deficits that emerge during the premorbid phase, worsen in the prodromal phase, and fully develop after the onset of the disorder (Harvey & Isner, 2020). Individuals with childhood or adolescent onset experience more pronounced neurocognitive deficits, greater disabilities, and a higher prevalence of withdrawal and negative symptoms (Driver et al., 2020; Grover et al., 2019). A specific subgroup of adults with psychosis exhibits a predominance of negative symptoms and significant cognitive impairments, particularly in processing speed and attention (Zhang et al., 2024). Additionally, individuals experiencing psychosis may be distressed by their symptoms, further impairing their functioning and cognition. Therefore, cognitive decline in psychosis may arise directly from cognitive deficits inherent to the disorder or indirectly from the psychological distress caused by psychotic symptoms. It is crucial to determine the person's baseline cognitive level and assess any changes. Since a person's ability to manage everyday tasks and challenges does not always align with their cognitive abilities, the assessment of cognitive profiles should be accompanied by an evaluation of adaptive functions.

Assessment of Adaptive Behaviour

Adaptive functioning includes practical, social, and conceptual skills essential for independent living. Among the most commonly used scales for assessing adaptive behaviour in adults are the Vineland-3 (Vineland Adaptive Behaviour Scales, Version 3) (Sparrow et al., 2016) and the ABAS-3 (Adaptive Behaviour Assessment System) (Harrison & Oakland, 2015). Both scales are standardized and validated, encompassing measures of various aspects of social, communicative, and practical behaviour. The procedure is semi-structured and requires collecting information from informants with first-hand knowledge of the person, most commonly family members, professional caregivers, and teachers.

The Vineland-3 identifies strengths and weaknesses across three core domains: social, practical, and behavioural adaptation, with optional additional assessments for motor skills and maladaptive behaviour. The American version covers the entire lifespan, offering an interview form for parents/caregivers and questionnaires for parents and teachers (for ages 3–21), available in both comprehensive and brief formats (Sparrow et al., 2016). Results provide scores across five subdomains and a total adaptive behaviour score. The score is based on the most typical performance on a task, not the capability to do it under optimal circumstances. Skills that require prompting in different ways are not considered adaptive skills. Due to cultural differences in expected behaviour between American and Scandinavian children (Smith et al., 2006), a Scandinavian version covering ages 3–26 years has been developed, with an ongoing process to expand it to the entire age range (pearsonsclinical.no).

The ABAS-3 includes five rating forms, tailored by age and by raters: one for parents rating children ages 0–5, another for daycare providers for children ages 2–5, two forms for ages 5–21 (one for parents and one for teachers), and one for adults (ages 16–89). The forms should be completed by parents, family members, teachers, supervisors, or the user as a self-report. Behaviour is rated on a four-point scale indicating the frequency of each behaviour when needed. Scores are provided by skill area (10 different skills, rated from extremely low to high) with scaled scores (mean of 10, SD of 3). Overall scores include a general adaptive composite and conceptual, social, and practical domains, also reported in percentiles.

Although both the ABAS-3 and Vineland-3 systems classify the severity of intellectual disabilities according to the levels of support needed to achieve a person's optimal personal functioning, they differ slightly. Vineland-3 assesses what a person typically does, while ABAS-3 focuses on their capability and frequency of behaviour, highlighting strengths. ABAS-3 uses questionnaires, making it quicker to administer, while Vineland-3 requires a detailed interview, potentially increasing the accuracy of results. For assessing children and diagnosing autism, Vineland-3's motor domain can be valuable, which ABAS-3 lacks. Regarding both tools, results should be interpreted considering the person's developmental level, age, and cultural background. Interpretation is generally conducted by professionals such as psychologists, psychiatrists, social workers, or mental health nurses. The results must be considered within the context of the person's age and cultural background (Tassé et al., 2016).

Real-world adaptive skills are affected by neuropsychological performance, symptoms, and functional capacity. People with psychosis in community settings demonstrate widespread functional impairments regardless of their level of residential independence, affecting their ability to manage social interactions, personal care, and financial responsibilities even in controlled settings. According to Bowie and colleagues (2010), the relationship between adaptive life skills in real-world settings and psychosis is linked to lifelong impairments across various domains, particularly among young and middle-aged adults. This holds true even for people who respond to antipsychotic treatment and exhibit only residual psychotic symptoms. Functional impairments can affect social, occupational, and independent living activities. In clinical samples, people in outpatient settings often experience widespread functional impairments, regardless of their level of residential independence, which hinders their ability to manage social interactions, personal care, and financial responsibilities, even in controlled environments (Bowie et al., 2010).

Assessments of adaptive skills should take into account the coexistence of both limitations and strengths in each person, as personalized, ongoing support can significantly enhance overall functioning and quality of life. Bridging the gap between cognitive and adaptive skills requires tailored strategies informed by assessment results. These strategies empower individuals to navigate daily tasks and challenges more effectively. For example, incorporating technological aids, such as visual supports or specialized applications, can enhance cognitive functioning and adaptability.

Emotional Development

Emotional development encompasses the understanding and management of emotions, including how they arise, our awareness of them, their significance, and how we regulate and express them. Behaviour is strongly connected to emotional development, and a person's level of emotional functioning plays an essential role in shaping their well-being, behaviour, and relationships. Because emotional dysregulation often does not align with cognitive abilities or adaptive skills, assessing this domain provides valuable insights for creating effective habilitation or rehabilitation plans, as well as therapeutic relationships with professional caregivers.

Emotional Functioning in Intellectual Disabilities

Level of emotional development is closely linked to the severity of intellectual disabilities, with those having comorbid autism exhibiting even lower levels of emotional development (Sappok et al., 2020). Although challenging behaviour is not part of the diagnosis of intellectual disabilities, it can be frequent, intense, and sometimes pose a threat to themselves or others (Lloyd & Kennedy, 2014). Interestingly, challenging behaviour is more closely correlated with the level of emotional development than with IQ. Furthermore, the type of challenging behaviour varies and depends on the person's level of emotional development. Aggression toward oneself and isolation are more prevalent at the lowest emotional levels, while aggression toward objects and other people is more common in emotional functioning between 6 and 18 months (Hermann et al., 2022). While individuals with intellectual disabilities may temporarily manage various situations, their behaviour may regress under prolonged stress or overwhelming situations, such as psychosis or other mental health conditions (Barrett et al., 2024).

Emotional Functioning in Psychosis

In people with psychosis without intellectual disabilities, severe dysfunction in emotion regulation may be observed (Berglund et al., 2023; Khoury & Lecomte, 2012). Furthermore, emotional dysregulation is associated with negative clinical outcomes, including exacerbated symptoms and social difficulties (Bartolomeo et al., 2022). Studies suggest that people with psychosis often regulate emotions inefficiently, over-regulating in low-stress situations and under-regulating in high-stress ones (Bartolomeo et al., 2022). Some people may display conduct disorder traits in childhood, while others develop challenging behaviour at the onset of psychosis (Hodgins, 2022).

Emotional Development and Tailored Treatment

When interventions do not align with a person's emotional level, they may provoke negative emotions and behaviours. Thus, a clear understanding of a person's level of emotional development is crucial; without it, there is a significant risk of developing ineffective or even harmful intervention plans. Adopting a developmental perspective offers vital insights, as specific behavioural patterns often correspond to distinct emotional developmental stages. Misinterpreting these behaviours as mere attention-seeking or boundary-testing can lead to ineffective interventions and inadequate support, causing increased symptoms. This may, in turn, result in chronic challenging behaviour (Emerson et al., 2001).

Tailoring interventions based on emotional development, along with environmental adjustments and staff training, has proven effective in reducing challenging behaviour. Assessing and adapting support based on emotional development, such as environmental adjustments and staff training, can reduce psychotropic medication use in persons with intellectual disabilities and challenging behaviour (Barrett et al., 2024). Additionally, recognizing specific behavioural patterns that align with particular emotional reference age groups may help differentiate between challenging behaviour and psychopathological symptoms (Hermann et al., 2022). By identifying emotional levels, professionals can differentiate between challenging behaviour stemming from developmental delays and behaviours arising from psychotic symptoms, allowing for more accurate and supportive interventions (Hermann et al., 2022).

SEED-2—A Measure of Emotional Development

The SEED-2 assessment tool can help distinguish whether behaviours arise from intellectual disabilities or psychosis, and identify psychotic symptoms unique to psychosis. The SEED-2 is a semi-structured tool that assesses the level of emotional development. It is based on Anton Dosen's model of emotional development, which integrates insights from different developmental domains: psychosocial development, attachment, and self-identity. The model highlights the risk of sensory and emotional overload in persons with intellectual disabilities, noting that intense stress can exacerbate maladaptive behaviours—such as stereotypies, self-harm, and restlessness—which may indicate stress reactions or underlying mental health conditions (Dosen, 2005a, 2005b).

SEED-2 encompasses emotional stages from 0 to 18 years (Tarasova et al., 2022), and it is applicable for measuring emotional levels in persons with borderline intellectual disabilities, dementia, and conditions beyond intellectual disabilities/autism spectrum disorder. The assessment involves interviews with at least two persons who know the individual well in different contexts and may include direct observations. It includes 140 questions across the following emotional domains: body awareness, orientation to the primary caregiver, reactions to surroundings, differentiation of feelings, peer relationships, interaction with the material world, communication, and emotion regulation. The emotional domains are assessed across six developmental levels, each linked to specific emotional behaviours, themes, and basic needs: the neonatal phase (0–6 months), the socialization phase (7–18 months), the autonomy and first individuation phase (19–36 months), the identification/ego-formation phase (4–7 years), emerging reality awareness (8–12 years), and social individuation (13–18 years). The last phase marks the transition to adulthood, characterized by social and personal maturation, indicating mild to borderline intellectual disabilities.

Although SEED-2 is not a diagnostic tool, it offers insights into a person's behaviour, needs, and motivations, helping to develop tailored supportive strategies. The tool enhances understanding for caregivers and professionals, using straightforward language to translate complex clinical concepts into everyday terms. This approach bridges the gap between specialized knowledge and the person's real-life experiences, fostering a common language for discussing emotional development. An individual intervention plan should be based on the results of this comprehensive assessment, providing a clearer picture of the person's strengths and needs. This approach facilitates tailored interventions that enhance quality of life, set realistic goals, and allow for ongoing development and necessary adjustments.

Conclusive Remarks

A comprehensive understanding of a person's adaptive abilities, and emotional level of development, is essential for the personalized adaptation of treatment plans. A lack of awareness of cognitive difficulties may limit opportunities for growth and hinder the realization of potential. Identifying both strengths and weaknesses is critical for designing targeted training and support. By distinguishing between persistent difficulties that require long-term habilitation and temporary challenges that benefit from short-term interventions, detailed and effective treatment plans can be developed. Person-specific tailored interventions have the potential to promote meaningful progress.

References

American Psychiatric Association, APA. (2013). Cautionary statement for forensic use of DSM-5. *Diagnostic and statistical manual of mental disorders* (5th ed.).

Barrett, B. F., Wehmeyer, M., Kolb, J., Ostermann, T., & Sappok, T. (2024). Impact of the emotional development approach on psychotropic medication in adults with intellectual and developmental disabilities: A retrospective clinical analysis. *Journal of Intellectual Disability Research.*

Bartolomeo, L. A., Raugh, I. M., & Strauss, G. P. (2022). Deconstructing emotion regulation in schizophrenia: The nature and consequences of abnormalities in monitoring dynamics. *Schizophrenia Research, 240*, 135–142.

Berglund, A. M., James, S. H., Raugh, I. M., & Strauss, G. P. (2023). Beliefs about the uncontrollability and usefulness of emotion in the schizophrenia-spectrum: Links to emotion regulation and negative symptoms. *Cognitive Therapy and Research, 47*(2), 282–294.

Bowie, C. R., Reichenberg, A., Patterson, T. L., Heaton, R. K., & Harvey, P. D. (2010). Determinants of real-world functional performance in psychosis subjects: Correlations with cognition, functional capacity, and symptoms. *Focus, 8*(4), 638–646.

Dosen, A. (2005a). Applying the developmental perspective in the psychiatric assessment and diagnosis of persons with intellectual disability: Part I—Assessment. *Journal of Intellectual Disability Research, 49*(1), 1–8.

Dosen, A. (2005b). Applying the developmental perspective in the psychiatric assessment and diagnosis of persons with intellectual disability: Part II—Diagnosis. *Journal of Intellectual Disability Research, 49*(1), 9–15.

Driver, D., Thomas, S., Gogtay, N., & Rapaport, J. L. (2020). Childhood-onset psychosis and early-onset psychosis spectrum disorders: An update. *Child and Adolescent Psychiatric Clinics of North America, 29*(1), 71–90.

Emerson, E., Kiernan, C., Alborz, A., Reeves, D., Mason, H., Swarbrick, R., Mason, L., & Hatton, C. (2001). The prevalence of challenging behaviours: A total population study. *Research in Developmental Disabilities, 22*(1), 77–93.

Grover, S., Sahoo, S., & Nehra, R. (2019). A comparative study of childhood/adolescent and adult-onset psychosis: Does the neurocognitive and psychosocial outcome differ? *Asian Journal of Psychiatry, 43*, 160–169.

Harrison, P. L., & Oakland, T. (2015). Adaptive behaviour assessment system. In C. Henington, & T. Wu (Eds.). *Mental measurements yearbook* (3rd ed.).

Harvey, P. D., & Isner, E. C. (2020). Cognition, social cognition, and functional capacity in early-onset psychosis. *Child and Adolescent Psychiatric Clinics of North America, 29*(1), 171–182.

Hermann, H., Berndt, N., Lytochkin, A., & Sappok, T. (2022). Behavioural phenomena in persons with an intellectual developmental disorder according to the level of emotional development. *Journal of Intellectual Disability Research, 66*(5), 483–498.

Hodgins, S. (2022). Could expanding and investing in first-episode psychosis services prevent aggressive behaviour and violent crime? *Frontiers in Psychiatry, 13*, Article 821760.

Khoury, B., & Lecomte, T. (2012). Emotion regulation and schizophrenia. *International Journal of Cognitive Therapy, 5*(1), 67–76.

Lloyd, B. P., & Kennedy, C. H. (2014). Assessment and treatment of challenging behaviour for persons with intellectual disability: A research review. *Journal of Applied Research in Intellectual Disabilities, 27*(3), 187–199.

Pearson Clinical. (2024, July 25). www.pearsonclinical.no

Sappok, T., Heinrich, M., & Böhm, J. (2020). The impact of emotional development in people with autism spectrum disorder and intellectual developmental disability. *Journal of Intellectual Disability Research, 64*(12), 946–955.

Smelror, R. E., & Ueland, T. (2023). In I. Agarts, & R. E. Smelror (Eds.), *Adolescent psychosis. Clinical and scientific perspectives.* Elsevier Academic press.

Smith, T., Eikeseth, S., & Lande, H. (2006). The Vineland adaptive behaviour scale in a sample of Norwegian second-grade children: A preliminary study. *Tidsskrift for Norsk Psykologforening, 43*(10), 1036–1039.

Sparrow, S. S., Cicchetti, D. V., & Saulnier, C. A. (2016). *Vineland adaptive behaviour scales* (3rd ed.). Pearson Assessments.

Tarasova, D., Zepperitz, S., Ronsse, E., Vonk, J., Zaal, S., Hudson, M., & Sappok, T. (2022). Social individuation: Extending the scale of emotional development—Short (SED-S) for adolescent reference ages. *Research in Developmental Disabilities, 128*, Article 104303.

Tassé, M. J., Luckasson, R., & Schalock, R. L. (2016). The relation between intellectual functioning and adaptive behaviour in the diagnosis of intellectual disability. *Intellectual and Developmental Disabilities, 54*(6), 381–390.

Zhang, T., Wei, Y., Tang, X., et al. (2024). Cognitive impairments in drug-naive patients with first-episode negative symptom–dominant psychosis. *JAMA Network Open, 7*(6), e2415110.

6

Biological Aspects, Pharmacology, and Adverse Effects

Jacopo Santambrogio and Emma Francia

Abstract Psychosis arises from a complex interaction between genetic and environmental factors. Knowledge about biological aspects is paramount for professionals who provide mental health services to people with intellectual disabilities who develop psychosis. This chapter includes core biological aspects: aetiology, comorbid intellectual disabilities and psychosis, and additional physical and mental health conditions, psychopharmacology, and adverse effects from antipsychotic medication. A case study will illustrate how a combination of conventional diagnostic assessment based on symptoms and impaired functioning along with newer insights into the biological aspects of psychosis can facilitate diagnostic work and effective treatment.

J. Santambrogio (✉)
Azienda Socio Sanitaria Territoriale della Brianza, Limbiate, Italy
e-mail: jacopo.santambrogio@asst-brianza.it

E. Francia
Milan, Italy

T. L. Bakken (ed.), *Psychosis in Adolescents and Adults with Intellectual Disabilities*,
https://doi.org/10.1007/978-3-031-95318-7_6

Keywords Aetiology · Co-morbidity · Psychopharmacology · Adverse effects · The UKU SERS-ID

Aetiology

Research on psychosis indicate that the condition is caused by complex and heterogeneous interactions between various biopsychosocial factors, including genetic, perinatal, neuroanatomic, neurochemical, and other biological factors (Ayano, 2016). This means that the pathophysiology of psychosis requires a broader understanding. The ancient concept of "dementia praecox" (Jablensky et al., 1993), which suggested that people with psychosis went through a slow progressive decline after normal development, underpinned the view of psychosis as a neurodegenerative condition with onset in early adulthood. In more recent years, there has been a shift towards a neurodevelopmental model of psychosis, implying that psychosis could result from inadequate development of the nervous system.

Genome-wide association studies have provided experimental evidence that will improve understanding of the genetic models and biological risk factors involved in this condition. These studies have discovered uncommon copy number variations (CNVs) and common single nucleotide polymorphisms with alleles associated with psychosis (Gejman et al., 2010). Epidemiological studies have highlighted a shared genetic risk for lower IQ and psychosis, with the strength of the genetic effects increasing with decreased IQ (Smeland et al., 2020). Neurodevelopmental genes identified in psychosis include genes involved in cell growth and behaviour regulation, such as DISC1, NRG1, DTNBP1, KCNH2, AKT1, PAK7, and RGS4 (Harrison & Weinberger, 2005; Korb & Hassiotis, 2022; Ng et al., 2009).

Results from imaging studies support a model that considers psychosis to be a result of disturbed early development of the nervous system. While the genetic component is considerable, with reported heritability estimates of up to 80%, environmental stressors are also implicated in the development of psychosis, such as childhood trauma, maternal immune infection, obstetric complications, and cannabis use. However, the effects of these stressors in psychosis are assumed to be mediated by epigenetic mechanisms.

The association between intellectual disabilities and psychosis may be a function of a severe and early-onset form of psychosis rather than the pre-existing intellectual disabilities themselves acting as a risk factor for the development of psychosis (Bonnici et al., 2007). Other theories hypothesize that low IQ in itself may involve a risk of psychosis, which could explain the significantly increased risk of psychosis in people with intellectual disabilities (Bakken et al., 2024b). For example, one hypothesis is that cognitive deficits in processing information, problem-solving, and planning, as well as emotional and social deficits, increase a person's vulnerability to psychosis (Korb & Hassiotis, 2022; Smeland et al., 2020).

Associations between intellectual disabilities and psychosis can be found in some genetic syndromes, such as the 22q11.2 deletion syndrome (also referred to as Di George syndrome or velocardiofacial syndrome), which is caused by the deletion of a small region of DNA on the long arm of chromosome 22 (Santambrogio et al., 2020). One percent of people with psychosis are estimated to have this mutation (Bassett et al., 2010), and psychosis develops in up to about 40% of those affected by the syndrome (Schneider et al., 2014).

For many decades, psychiatrists and neurologists thought that people with intellectual disabilities could not suffer from mental health conditions. This theory was based on the concept that intellectual disabilities are caused by biological factors, either genetic or traumatic, resulting in brain injury. According to this theory, a "graft-psychosis" could arise in early adulthood, manifesting particularly as challenging behaviour. In these cases, antipsychotics were the pharmacological treatment of choice. Psychiatrists have only recently become more conscious of and sensitive to the question of mental health in people with intellectual disabilities, recognizing that they are particularly vulnerable to mental health conditions throughout their neurodevelopmental process.

Co-morbidity

Psychosis is currently viewed as being caused by complex and heterogeneous interactions between various biopsychosocial factors. This view is supported by the increased risk of co-occurring physical conditions, poor physical health, and early death in people with psychosis (Andreassen et al., 2023; Grant et al., 2022; Santambrogio et al., 2023; Zhang et al., 2022). Consequently, life expectancy is estimated to be about 15 years less than that of the general population (Grant et al., 2022). A Swedish register study found that people with intellectual disabilities and psychosis had significantly higher prevalence of cardiovascular disorders, digestive disorders, and obesity and metabolic disorders compared to both the general population and people with psychosis without cognitive impairments (Bakken et al., submitted). Cardiovascular diseases are generally found to be a major cause of poor physical health in people with psychosis (Veeneman et al., 2022). An international register study of physical health in people with psychosis found a high risk for co-morbidity in the respiratory, gastrointestinal, and liver systems (Mulugeta et al., 2023). Higher rates of obesity, metabolic syndrome, and diabetes are also associated with psychosis (Suvisaari et al., 2016). Newer generation antipsychotic medications, such as Clozapine and Olanzapine, are particularly associated with weight gain and obesity. Annamalai et al. (2017) compared people treated for psychosis with a control group from the general population and found that obesity occurred twice as often in the people with psychosis. In the same study, diabetes was found about three times as often in the people with psychosis compared to the controls in the general population.

People with both intellectual disabilities and psychosis may have an especially high risk of co-morbidities. However, the risk of the co-morbidities described above in people diagnosed with psychosis has not been extensively studied in people with intellectual disabilities, as they rarely participate in mental health studies (Camanni et al., 2021).

Epilepsy associated with psychosis is worth special attention. Psychotic episodes may occur in epilepsy, but they rarely reflect the presence of a chronic psychotic condition. In other cases, the relationship between epileptic seizures and psychotic episodes is one of alternating events (forced normalization) (Beghi et al., 2010a). Moreover, antipsychotic medications can lower the seizure threshold, so a person with intellectual disabilities and psychosis could experience epileptic seizures due to antipsychotic treatment, which may need to be reduced or changed (Beghi et al., 2010b).

Psychopharmacology

Recommendations for antipsychotic medication for people with concurrent intellectual disabilities and psychosis usually follow the guidelines for others suffering from psychosis, with necessary adaptations for people with intellectual disabilities (Humphries et al., 2020). However, research on antipsychotic medications for people with intellectual disabilities is still not at the randomized controlled trial (RCT) level (Ayub et al., 2015). There is a lack of studies comparing specific antipsychotics for people with intellectual disabilities, to those in the general population, or comparing different antipsychotics in RCTs (Deb et al., 2023b). One reason for this knowledge gap is that intellectual disabilities itself may be an exclusion criterion in RCTs (Camanni et al., 2021). Most published studies on antipsychotic drugs for people with intellectual disabilities include clinical samples, such as Bakken et al. (2007).

A considerable concern regarding antipsychotic medication for people with intellectual disabilities is the off-label use to reduce challenging behaviour (de Kuijper et al., 2010; Deb et al., 2023a; Sheehan & Hassiotis, 2017; Song et al., 2020). These studies highlight the need for more research on the off-label use of antipsychotic medication. The effectiveness of this use is also questionable (de Kuijper et al., 2010; Deb et al., 2023a; Sheehan & Hassiotis, 2017). In fact, studies have shown that the use of antipsychotics to manage challenging behaviour in people with intellectual disabilities has sparse evidence. On the contrary, off-label use of antipsychotics could cause harmful adverse effects (Sheehan & Hassiotis, 2017). In a randomized controlled trial from 2008, published in The Lancet, risperidone and haloperidol were compared to placebo in the treatment of aggressive behaviour in people with intellectual disabilities (Tyrer et al., 2008). After 4 weeks of treatment, the placebo group did not differ from the risperidone or haloperidol groups regarding the effect on behaviour that challenges.

Despite evidence supporting the discontinuation of off-label use of antipsychotics for people with intellectual disabilities, it may be difficult to scale down and eventually discontinue this medication. De Kuijper and Hoekstra investigated the discontinuation of off-label use of antipsychotics in a large Dutch community sample (2017). Of the sample of 3299 people with intellectual disabilities, 977 used antipsychotics, which is 30%. Reasons for physicians not to discontinue the use of antipsychotics in those who used off-label antipsychotics for more than one year included concerns about symptoms of restlessness, a diagnosis of autism spectrum disorder, previously unsuccessful discontinuation, and/or objections from legal representatives or staff. There was high variability in reasons among the participating physicians. The off-label use included old-generation antipsychotics such as Chlorpromazine, Zuclopenthixol, Levomepromazine, Promazine, Haloperidol, and Clotiapine. Most of the use was conducted without assessing a proper diagnosis of psychosis (de Kuijper et al., 2010).

A diagnosis of psychosis should be confirmed by clinical assessment and test evaluations before prescribing antipsychotic treatment for people with intellectual disabilities, as well as for those with autism spectrum disorders. An Italian tool, the Systematic Psychopathological Assessment for those with Intellectual and Developmental Disabilities—General screening (SPAIDD-G, Bertelli, 2019), which provides diagnostic orientations including psychosis, could be helpful.

An English project, STOMP, was established to facilitate the reduction of off-label use of antipsychotics, with the same arguments as in De Kuijper and Hoekstra (2017), and Tyrer and colleagues (2008). STOMP (Shankar et al., 2019) concluded that there are pitfalls to avoid when reducing or discontinuing antipsychotics in people with intellectual disabilities. The first pitfall is overlooking an unrecognized mental health condition, such as psychosis. Hence, an assessment of possible mental health conditions should be conducted parallel to the reduction of medication. It could be that the behaviour that caused the use of antipsychotics in the first place was, in fact, atypical symptoms of psychosis. The second pitfall is misinterpreting confounding symptoms of physical pain or psychological or social challenges, such as a career change or losing a parent. Also, multi-morbidity of both physical and mental health conditions, including physical pain and neurocognitive conditions, is associated with challenging behaviour. Considering that some antipsychotics are used as analgesics or even sedatives for sleep, the aforementioned conditions should also be ruled out.

Atypical antipsychotics such as Risperidone, Paliperidone, Quetiapine, Olanzapine, Aripiprazole, Lurasidone, Cariprazine, Brexpiprazole, and Clozapine are commonly used to treat psychosis in people with intellectual disabilities and seem to be better tolerated than those of previous generations (Advokat et al., 2000). Specific focus is needed for Clozapine, which is effective for treatment-resistant psychosis and is safe and efficacious for people with intellectual disabilities (Marconi & Martin, 2024; Rohde et al., 2018; Thalayasingam et al., 2004). As stated by Ayub and colleagues in a review published by the Cochrane Library, there were no specific RCTs about Clozapine in an ID population until 2015 (Ayub et al., 2015), and urgent research is still needed on this topic. Only one protocol regarding an ongoing RCT in Spain has been published to date (Alemany-Navarro et al., 2024).

When symptoms have been stabilized, there may be a need further prophylactic treatment to reduce the risk of relapse, and discontinuation of antipsychotic medication may involve a poorer prognosis compared to those who are provided with prophylactic pharmacotherapy to prevent relapse (Hui et al., 2018).

"Daniel"

Daniel is a 32-year-old male with moderate intellectual disabilities, an IQ of 57, and low adaptive behaviour. He is diagnosed with psychosis. He is overweight and has an accelerated pulse rate, although his cerebral MRI is normal. Born after a normal pregnancy, Daniel showed motor delays early on. He was bullied at school, which he attended with the support of a special needs teacher. He was admitted to a mental health institution for minors after developing behaviours that challenge, such as stealing money from his parents, leaving home at night without reason, and wandering through town. On one occasion, he jumped from a window due to psychotic symptoms, likely hearing voices. When first responders arrived, they took him to the emergency room. He was upset and his speech was unintelligible and fragmented, expressing fears such as having cancer and failing because he did not get a driving license.

His parents described paranoid thoughts and behaviours, such as accusing them of damaging his life, social withdrawal, apathy, and occasional aggressiveness. He was also reported to talk to himself, likely hearing voices, and alternately crying and laughing. Behaviourally, his adaptive behaviour remains low; he can only manage some gardening tasks and struggles with managing money when asked to do shopping. He has been treated with Risperidone, Gabapentin, and Delorazepam, with Promazine as needed, since he was 17. Sometimes he refuses to take his medication. His mother, who suffers from both a neurological illness and a mental disorder, shows high levels of anger and criticism towards Daniel, referring to him as "a column that speaks, he is not a human being anymore, I am scared he becomes chronic."

His parents, now separated, sought help from the local outpatient service and a consultant psychiatrist to find a protected mental health institute due to the difficulties in caring for their son at home. In 2021, Daniel was finally hospitalized in a rehabilitative mental health facility. His treatment was changed, with Risperidone (due to its sedative effects and hyperprolactinemia) being substituted with Clozapine and Lurasidone, which improved his impulsiveness and anxiety. By 2024, he still has some paranoid thoughts, but when he talks to himself, he laughs instead of crying, suggesting the voices are more friendly. He shows acquiescence when answering questions. Additionally, he has started a diet for obesity, and his physical issues are being addressed. He participates in educational and social activities, such as swimming lessons, which he enjoys and excels at. Overall, his quality of life is slightly improving.

As illustrated in the case above, diagnostic assessment of psychosis in people with intellectual disabilities is currently based on the interpretation of symptoms and social functioning. However, recent research hypothesizes that biological measurements and medical diagnostic tests may become a more important part of the assessment process

(Andreassen et al., 2023). A study published in 2020 involving about 80,000 people diagnosed with psychosis indicates an association between lower intelligence and psychosis, while no such association was found for bipolar disorder (Smeland et al., 2020).

Adverse Effects

Monitoring adverse effects, also known as side effects, is crucial (Tveter et al., 2016), as people with intellectual disabilities may have difficulty reporting them. For instance, tardive dyskinesia may be more common among this population (Fodstad et al., 2010). Monitoring adverse effects from antipsychotic medication is also important because they can easily be mistaken for symptoms of mental illness, or vice versa. Features of akathisia (restlessness, inability to sit still), a common side effect of antipsychotic medications such as aripiprazole, may also be observed in people with anxiety (Bakken et al., 2024a, 2024b). In such cases, proper differential diagnosis is necessary. If akathisia is identified as an antipsychotic side effect, the medication should be reduced and supplemented with a benzodiazepine. Tardive dyskinesia and unusual motor movements can also be confused.

When systematically evaluating the treatment effects and adverse effects of antipsychotics, it is essential to establish a baseline prior to initiating treatment (Humphries et al., 2020; Tveter et al., 2016). Guidelines recommend regular monitoring of blood glucose, lipids, and weight for people taking antipsychotic medications to prevent the risk of diabetes, hypercholesterolemia, and metabolic syndromes in general. Clozapine requires specific follow-up with blood tests due to the risk of inducing potentially fatal agranulocytosis. Persons with early-onset psychosis who are diagnosed with autism spectrum disorder may have an increased tendency for antipsychotic treatment failure. About 50% of participants in a study investigating psychosis treatment in people with autism spectrum disorders switched their first antipsychotic drug due to intolerable side effects (Downs et al., 2017).

The UKU Side effect rating Scale for Adults with Intellectual Disabilities (UKU-SERS-ID) is an useful instrument for monitoring potential side effects in people with intellectual disabilities who are receiving psychopharmacological treatment (Bakken et al., 2024a, 2024b; Tveter et al., 2016). It was developed to detect side effects among people with intellectual disabilities in inpatient mental health settings. The reliability and validity of the UKU-SERS-ID have been found to be good to acceptable (Tveter et al., 2016). The UKU SERS-ID is feasible in clinical practice and should be scored by nurses or other health professionals and then interpreted by a medical doctor (Bakken et al., 2024a, 2024b).

It is important to gather information from multiple sources when evaluating treatment and possible side effects (Rysstad et al., 2022). Since mental health professionals may not have a comprehensive overview of the person's previous functioning, clinicians depend on information from family members and/or professional caregivers to make appropriate judgments when evaluating treatment.

Conclusive Remarks

The new knowledge about biological factors in mental health, particularly concerning people with intellectual disabilities, should prompt clinicians to incorporate this understanding into their assessments and treatments. Certain genetic syndromes, especially 22q11 deletion syndrome, are associated with a high risk of developing psychosis. Therefore, clinicians should be aware of this heightened risk. Additionally, the high risk of co-morbidity, both mental and physical, should be considered.

Antipsychotic medication is frequently used to reduce behaviour that challenges, although the scientific evidence supporting this use is quite limited. Considering the potential side effects and the difficulties associated with reducing and discontinuing antipsychotics, a thorough assessment of other explanations for behaviour that challenges should be conducted before prescribing antipsychotics. Monitoring for side effects should always be performed when people with intellectual disabilities are prescribed antipsychotics.

The evidence for the use of antipsychotic medication in treating psychosis in people with intellectual disabilities remains sparse. However, clinical studies have shown that multimodal interventions, including antipsychotics, can be effective. Nonetheless, there is still a need for more research on psychopharmacology, particularly randomized controlled trials. Studies that include both people with and without intellectual disabilities who are diagnosed with psychosis are needed and desired.

References

Advokat, C. D., Mayville, E. A., & Matson, J. L. (2000). Side effect profiles of atypical antipsychotics, typical antipsychotics, or no psychotropic medications in persons with mental retardation. *Research in Developmental Disabilities, 21*(1), 75–84.

Alemany-Navarro, M., Sánchez-Barbero, B., Reguera-Pozuelo, P., Altea-Manzano, L., Gómez-Garrido, A., Rocha-González, I., Ruiz Veguilla, M., & Crespo-Facorro, B. (2024). Efficacy of clozapine versus standard treatment in adult persons with intellectual disability and treatment-resistant psychosis (CLOZAID): Study protocol of a multicenter randomized clinical trial. *Frontiers in Psychiatry, 15*, 1400621.

Andreassen, O. A., Hindley, G. F., Frei, O., & Smeland, O. B. (2023). New insights from the last decade of research in psychiatric genetics: Discoveries, challenges and clinical implications. *World Psychiatry, 22*(1), 4–24.

Annamalai, A., Kosir, U., & Tek, C. (2017). Prevalence of obesity and diabetes in patients with schizophrenia. *World Journal of Diabetes, 8*(8), 390.

Ayano, G. (2016). Schizophrenia: A concise overview of etiology, epidemiology diagnosis and management: Review of literatures. *J Schizophrenia Res, 3*(2), 2–7.

Ayub, M., Saeed, K., Munshi, T. A., & Naeem, F. (2015). Clozapine for psychotic disorders in adults with intellectual disabilities. *Cochrane Database of Systematic Reviews*, (9).

Bakken, T. L., Axmon, A., & Sandberg, M. (submitted). Co-morbidities in people with intellectual disability with schizophrenia compared to those with intellectual disability without schizophrenia, and schizophrenia without intellectual disability: A Swedish register study (IDcare).

Bakken, T. L., Hellerud, J. M. A., Skaale, S. E., Augustin, M., & Elvehaug, A. H. (2024a). The use of the UKU side effect rating scale for adults with intellectual disabilities in a clinical sample. *Advances in Mental Health and Intellectual Disabilities*.

Bakken, T. L., Sandberg, M., & Axmon, A. (2024b). Schizophrenia in children, adults and older people with intellectual disability compared with the general population: A Swedish register study (IDcare). *General Psychiatry, 37*(6).

Bassett, A. S., Scherer, S. W., & Brzustowicz, L. M. (2010). Copy number variations in schizophrenia: Critical review and new perspectives on concepts of genetics and disease. *American Journal of Psychiatry, 167*(8), 899–914.

Beghi, et al. (2010a). Psychiatric events associated with epilepsy | Gli eventi psichiatrici in corso di epilessia. *Quaderni Italiani di Psichiatria, 29*(3), 95–105.

Beghi, et al. (2010b). Current use of electroencephalography in patients with psychoses | Utilizzo dell'elettroencefalografia nelle psicosi oggi. *Quaderni Italiani di Psichiatria, 29*(4), 165–171.

Bertelli, M. O. (2019). *SPAIDD-G systematic psychopathological assessment for persons with intellectual and developmental disabilities—General screening.* Manuale, Giunti Psychometrics S.r.l.

Bonnici, H. M., William, T., Moorhead, J., Stanfield, A. C., Harris, J. M., Owens, D. G., Johnstone, E. C., & Lawrie, S. M. (2007). Pre-frontal lobe gyrification index in schizophrenia, mental retardation and comorbid groups: An automated study. *Neuroimage, 35*(2), 648–654.

Camanni, G., Ciccone, O., Lepri, A., Tinarelli, C., Menna, M., Baglioni, A., Murgia, N., & Elisei, S. (2021). Intellectual disability and psychiatric disorders as exclusion criteria in randomized controlled trials (RCT). *Psychiatria Danubina, 33*(suppl 11), 36–39.

De Kuijper, G. M., & Hoekstra, P. J. (2017). Physicians' reasons not to discontinue long-term used off-label antipsychotic drugs in people with intellectual disability. *Journal of Intellectual Disability Research, 61*(10), 899–908.

de Kuijper, G., Hoekstra, P., Visser, F., Scholte, F. A., Penning, C., & Evenhuis, H. (2010). Use of antipsychotic drugs in persons with intellectual disability (ID) in the Netherlands: Prevalence and reasons for prescription. *Journal of Intellectual Disability Research, 54*(7), 659–667.

Deb, S., Roy, M., & Limbu, B. (2023a). Pharmacological management of psychopathology in people with intellectual disabilities and/or autism spectrum disorder. *Bjpsych Advances, 29*(5), 322–333.

Deb, S., Roy, M., Limbu, B., Brizard, B. A., Murugan, M., Roy, A., & Santambrogio, J. (2023b). Randomised controlled trials of antipsychotics for people with autism spectrum disorder: A systematic review and a meta-analysis. *Psychological Medicine, 53*(16), 7964–7972.

Downs, J. M., Lechler, S., Dean, H., Sears, N., Patel, R., Shetty, H., Simonoff, E., Hotopf, M., Ford, T. J., Diaz-Caneja, C. M., Arango, C., MacCabe, J. H., Hayes, R. D., & Pina-Camacho, L. (2017). The association between comorbid autism spectrum disorders and antipsychotic treatment failure in early-onset psychosis: A historical cohort study using electronic health records. *The Journal of Clinical Psychiatry, 78*(9), 1411.

Fodstad, J. C., Bamburg, J. W., Matson, J. L., Mahan, S., Hess, J. A., Neal, D., & Holloway, J. (2010). Tardive dyskinesia and intellectual disability: An examination of demographics and topography in adults with dual diagnosis and atypical antipsychotic use. *Research in Developmental Disabilities, 31*(3), 750–759.

Gejman, P. V., Sanders, A. R., & Duan, J. (2010). The role of genetics in the etiology of schizophrenia. *Psychiatric Clinics, 33*(1), 35–66.

Grant, R. K., Brindle, W. M., Donnelly, M. C., McConville, P. M., Stroud, T. G., Bandieri, L., & Plevris, J. N. (2022). Gastrointestinal and liver disease in patients with schizophrenia: A narrative review. *World Journal of Gastroenterology, 28*(38), 5515.

Harrison, P. J., & Weinberger, D. R. (2005). Schizophrenia genes, gene expression, and neuropathology: On the matter of their convergence. *Molecular Psychiatry, 10*(1), 40–68.

Hui, C. L., Honer, W. G., Lee, E. H., Chang, W. C., Chan, S. K., Chen, E. S., Pang, E. P., Lui, S. S., Chung, D. W., Yeung, W. S., Ng, R. M., Lo, W. T., Jones, P. B., Sham, P., & Chen, E. Y. (2018). Long-term effects of discontinuation from antipsychotic maintenance following first-episode schizophrenia and related disorders: A 10 year follow-up of a randomised, double-blind trial. *The Lancet Psychiatry, 5*(5), 432–442.

Humphries, L., Michael, D., & Hassiotis, A. (2020). Schizophrenia and related psychoses in people with intellectual disability. *Oxford textbook of the psychiatry of intellectual disability* (pp. 91–104).

Jablensky, A., Hugler, H., Von Cranach, M., & Kalinov, K. (1993). Kraepelin revisited: A reassessment and statistical analysis of dementia praecox and manic-depressive insanity in 1908. *Psychological Medicine, 23*(4), 843–858.

Korb, L., & Hassiotis, A. (2022). Psychotic disorders. In M. O. Bertelli, S. S. Deb, K. Munir, A. Hassiotis, & L. Salvador-Carulla (Eds.), *Textbook of psychiatry for intellectual disability and autism spectrum disorder* (pp. 537–555). Springer International Publishing.

Marconi, A., & Martin, A. (2024). Navigating complexity: A case report on interplay of intellectual disability (ID), schizophrenia clozapine treatment and chemotherapy. *Bjpsych Open, 10*(S1), S282–S283.

Mulugeta, A., Suppiah, V., & Hyppönen, E. (2023). Schizophrenia and comorbidity risk: Evidence from a data driven phenomewide association study. *Journal of Psychiatric Research, 162*, 1–10.

Ng, M. Y. M., Levinson, D. F., Faraone, S. V., Suárez, B. K., DeLisi, L. E., Arinami, T., Riley, B., Paunio, T., Pulver, A. E., Irmansyah, Holmans, P. A., Escamilla, M., Wildenauer, D. B., Williams, N. M., Laurent, C., Mowry, B. J., Brzustowicz, L. M., Maziade, M., Sklar, P., … Lewis, C. M. (2009). Meta-analysis of 32 genome-wide linkage studies of schizophrenia. *Molecular Psychiatry, 14*(8), 774–785.

Rohde, C., Polcwiartek, C., Correll, C. U., & Nielsen, J. (2018). Real-World effectiveness of clozapine for intellectual disability: Results from a mirror-image and reverse-mirror-image study. *Journal of Psychopharmacology, 32*(11), 1197–1203.

Rysstad, A. L., Kildahl, A. N., Skavhaug, J. O., Dønnum, M. S., & Helverschou, S. B. (2022). Case study: Organizing outpatient pharmacological treatment of bipolar disorder in autism, intellectual disability and Phelan-McDermid syndrome (22q13. 3 deletion syndrome). *International Journal of Developmental Disabilities, 68*(3), 378–387.

Santambrogio, J., Bertelli, M. O., Terrevazzi, S., De Carolis, L., Francia, E., Boldoni, C., Calascibetta, M., Cudazzo, E., Lucca, C., Viganò, V., Danese, M., Minazzi, G. A., Santarone, A., Bianco, A., Hassiotis, A., & Clerici, M. (2023). Cognitive dysfunction and psychopathology: A cohort study of adults with intellectual developmental disorder. *Journal of Intellectual Disability Research, 67*(10), 1029–1045.

Santambrogio, J., Colmegna, F., Di Brita, C., Merra, A., Bertelli, M. O., & Clerici, M. (2020). Psychiatric and psychological support for an adolescent woman with chromosome 22 deletion syndrome and intellectual disability: A good outcome. *Rivista di Psichiatria, 55*(2), 106–111.

Schneider, M., Debbané, M., Bassett, A. S., Chow, E. W., Fung, W. L. A., Van Den Bree, M. B., Owen, M., Murphy, K. C., Niarchou, M., Kates, W. R., Antshel, K. M., Fremont, W., McDonald-McGinn, D. M., Gur, R. E., Zackai, E. H., Vorstman, J., Duijff, S. N., Klaassen, P. W. J., Swillen, A., … International Consortium on Brain and Behavior in 22q11. 2 Deletion Syndrome. (2014). Psychiatric disorders from childhood to adulthood in 22q11. 2 deletion syndrome: Results from the International Consortium on Brain and Behavior in 22q11. 2 Deletion Syndrome. *American Journal of Psychiatry, 171*(6), 627–639.

Sheehan, R., & Hassiotis, A. (2017). Reduction or discontinuation of antipsychotics for challenging behaviour in adults with intellectual disability: A systematic review. *The Lancet Psychiatry, 4*(3), 238–256.

Shankar, R., Wilcock, M., Oak, K., McGowan, P., & Sheehan, R. (2019). Stopping, rationalising or optimising antipsychotic drug treatment in people with intellectual disability and/or autism. *Drug and Therapeutics Bulletin, 57*(1), 10–13.

Smeland, O. B., Bahrami, S., Frei, O., Shadrin, A., O'Connell, K., Savage, J., Watanabe, K., Krull, F., Bettella, F., Steen, N. E., Ueland, T., Posthuma, D., Djurovic, S., Dale, A. M., & Andreassen, O. A. (2020). Genome-wide analysis reveals extensive genetic overlap between schizophrenia, bipolar disorder, and intelligence. *Molecular Psychiatry, 25*(4), 844–853.

Song, M., Ware, R., Doan, T. N., & Harley, D. (2020). Psychotropic medication use in adults with intellectual disability in Queensland, Australia, from 1999 to 2015: A cohort study. *Journal of Intellectual Disability Research, 64*(1), 45–56.

Suvisaari, J., Keinänen, J., Eskelinen, S., & Mantere, O. (2016). Diabetes and schizophrenia. *Current Diabetes Reports, 16*, 1–10.

Thalayasingam, S., Alexander, R. T., & Singh, I. (2004). The use of clozapine in adults with intellectual disability. *Journal of Intellectual Disability Research, 48*(6), 572–579.

Tveter, A. L., Bakken, T. L., Røssberg, J. I., Bech-Pedersen, E., & Bramness, J. G. (2016). Reliability and validity of the UKU side effect rating scale for adults with intellectual disabilities. *Advances in Mental Health and Intellectual Disabilities, 10*(3), 166–171.

Tyrer, P., Oliver-Africano, P. C., Ahmed, Z., Bouras, N., Cooray, S., Deb, S., Murphy, D., Hare, M., Meade, M., Reece, B., Kramo, K., Bhaumik, S., Harley, D., Regan, A., Thomas, D., Rao, B., North, B., Eliahoo, J., Karatela, S., … Crawford, M. (2008). Risperidone, haloperidol, and placebo in the treatment of aggressive challenging behaviour in patients with intellectual disability: A randomised controlled trial. *The Lancet, 371*(9606), 57–63.

Veeneman, R. R., Vermeulen, J. M., Abdellaoui, A., Sanderson, E., Wootton, R. E., Tadros, R., Bezzina, C. R., Denys, D., Munafò, M. R., Verweij, K. J. H., & Treur, J. L. (2022). Exploring the relationship between schizophrenia and cardiovascular disease: A genetic correlation and multivariable Mendelian randomization study. *Schizophrenia Bulletin, 48*(2), 463–473.

Zhang, R., Sjölander, A., Ploner, A., Lu, D., Bulik, C. M., & Bergen, S. E. (2022). Novel disease associations with schizophrenia genetic risk revealed in~ 400,000 UK Biobank participants. *Molecular Psychiatry, 27*(3), 1448–1454.

7

Psychosocial Interventions

Trine Lise Bakken

Abstract This chapter summarizes the knowledge about psychosocial interventions for persons with intellectual disabilities and psychosis. This is still an understudied topic, despite the long-term suffering of these people and their families. The effects of psychosocial interventions in psychosis remain unclear in people with intellectual disabilities, and there are no existing randomized controlled studies available. However, clinical studies have described psychosocial interventions and proven their effectiveness in smaller samples. These interventions include family interventions, individual and group therapy, sensory therapy aimed at reducing stress and anxiety, psychoeducation, and mental health nursing. Mental health nursing is an important psychosocial intervention, as it can be provided 24/7 and to the entire spectrum of people with intellectual disabilities.

T. L. Bakken (✉)
Oslo University Hospital, Oslo, Norway
e-mail: uxtlba@ous-hf.no

T. L. Bakken (ed.), *Psychosis in Adolescents and Adults with Intellectual Disabilities*,
https://doi.org/10.1007/978-3-031-95318-7_7

Keywords Relapse · Psychosocial intervention · Psychoeducation · Family interventions · Group therapy · Mental health nursing · Therapeutic communication · Emotional climate · Multiple complex needs

Combination Therapy

Even though psychopharmacological interventions are still the most studied interventions for psychosis, combination therapies—medication and psychosocial interventions—have proven to have better outcomes compared to medication alone (Guo et al., 2010). Guo and colleagues found that people receiving combination therapy had lower rates of discontinuation of treatment, lower relapse risk, and scored better on quality of life measures. Combination therapy is recommended for people with psychosis (van Os & Kapur, 2009), alongside a plan for crisis intervention (Birchwood et al., 2000). For people with intellectual disabilities and concurrent psychosis, inpatient admission in mental health services may be beneficial (Bakken & Martinsen, 2013). In acute phases, severe global functional deterioration and severely disorganized speech and behaviour may be observed, and the person may not be able to uphold basic self-care tasks such as eating, going to the bathroom, dressing, or maintaining social relationships (Bakken, 2014). Hence, a totally compensatory care system may be necessary. Elements from sensory therapy have been found to reduce stress and anxiety in persons admitted to mental health inpatient units (Andersen et al., 2017). See Chapter 8 for a thorough presentation of sensory therapy. Psychosocial interventions are also called adjuvant therapy, indicating psychopharmacological treatment is the main treatment. However, recent research indicates that in addition to psychopharmacological treatment, family interventions, psychoeducation, and cognitive therapy may be helpful when the person is no longer in an acute state dominated by fragmentation and anxiety (Bighelli et al., 2021).

A Norwegian clinical study found a range of psychosocial interventions provided for persons with psychosis and intellectual disabilities (Bakken et al., 2024). Bakken and colleagues studied treatment and interventions in a clinical sample in a nationwide study. One hundred and eighty-three adolescents and adults diagnosed with intellectual disabilities and autism spectrum disorder participated. Twenty-six, most of them with mild or moderate intellectual disabilities, were diagnosed with psychosis; all were provided with one or more psychopharmacological medications. Other interventions included inpatient admission, crisis management plans, family involvement, practical support, and training and supervision of community caregivers. Daily activities were also adjusted following the diagnosis of psychosis (Bakken et al., 2024).

People with psychosis may benefit from treatment in emergency units during acute phases. As mental health services and long-stay institutions for people with intellectual disabilities have been largely decentralized since the 1980s in Western countries, the length of stay in inpatient mental health services has decreased (Miguel & Helen, 2011). Multidisciplinary teams during assessment and treatment, including emergency inpatient settings in acute phases, rehabilitation, and long-term follow-up in community services, are recommended for people with intellectual disabilities and severe mental health conditions (Davis et al., 2008).

The Vulnerable Brain

Providing psychosocial interventions must take into account that people with intellectual disabilities, in addition to cognitive impairments, have weaker working memory and decreased capacity, which are among the factors contributing to vulnerable brains in people with intellectual disabilities. More recent research points to people with autism spectrum disorder, dementia, and other neurological conditions as being more likely to develop psychotic conditions than the general population (Gordon et al., 2016; Mulugeta et al., 2023). Hence, psychosis should be considered when people with intellectual disabilities show a severe decline in adaptive skills.

Two additional factors contribute to vulnerability in people with intellectual disabilities and may increase with co-morbid psychosis: sensory disintegration and cognitive overload. Sensory disintegration (difficulties with processing sensory information) occurs especially often in those with autism in addition to intellectual disabilities (Verhulst et al., 2022).

Anxiety reactions may be attributed to sensory over-responsivity. Experiences of sensory processing difficulties encompass all of the senses and may result in over- or under-reactivity to sensory inputs, which are useful for other people, like car horns (Kerstein, 2008). Cognitive overload may arise over time in people with intellectual disabilities when they experience stressful situations related to task-solving, sensory difficulties, or demanding social settings (Colvin & Sheehan, 2014). It is not a diagnostic category but a term for a "stressed brain." Some people with intellectual disabilities tend to perform better at speaking than at understanding what other people say, and consequently, their cognitive skills are overestimated. High-stress levels may cause acting out of emotional pain, which may be observed as temper tantrums and/or self-harm, often interpreted as psychosis in people with intellectual disabilities.

Support Persons in Individual and Group Therapy

One of the factors that differentiates mental health interventions for persons with intellectual disabilities from interventions in the general population is the need for a nurse or another professional caregiver alongside in individual or group therapy (Chester et al., 2020). Nursing staff spend more time with the person than other professionals like medical doctors or psychologists, and hence usually know the person's personal communication style better than the individual therapist, and the person usually feels safer with staff than with the individual therapist (Sommerstad et al., 2021). The mental health nurse may act as a facilitator and interpreter during the sessions. For persons who have not been to individual therapy before, the nursing staff may inform them about therapy, and in some cases, role-play may be a feasible preparation before starting individual sessions. Another important reason to have a nurse alongside in sessions is the need for an "external working memory," as intellectual disabilities and psychosis both negatively impact working memory (Bakken, 2021).

Psychoeducation

Psychoeducation involves basic education about mental health conditions, including coping with symptoms, communication, the risk of relapse, effects of treatment, prognosis, relapse prevention, and effects/side effects of antipsychotic medication (Bighelli et al., 2021). A meta-study including more than a thousand persons with psychosis found that the following interventions (in addition to medication) significantly reduced the risk of relapse: family interventions, family psychoeducation, and cognitive behavioural therapy. These treatments should be the first choice in the long-term treatment of psychosis. Psychoeducation for people with intellectual disabilities is still not studied in larger samples. However, psychoeducation for people with intellectual disabilities and additional mental health conditions has proven to be promising in clinical samples (Allott et al., 2013; Ashworth et al., 2017; Bakken et al., 2017; Crowley et al., 2008).

Family Interventions

Family involvement is crucial when caring for people with intellectual disabilities and mental health conditions (Bakken et al., 2017; Chester et al., 2020). However, families often report difficulties accessing services for their relatives with intellectual disabilities and mental health conditions, and collaborating with services may be experienced as challenging (Karlsen et al., 2024). As psychosis tends to be a long-lasting condition, causing considerable global functioning decline and multiple relapses, family interventions are essential. For example, psychoeducational multi-family groups (PMG) (McFarlane, 2016), may be adapted for people with intellectual disabilities and psychosis, and their families (Bakken et al., 2017). A clinical study investigated the participants' experiences of being part of such a group. Four participants with intellectual disabilities and psychosis, their close relatives, and community professional caregivers participated (Bakken et al., 2017). The participants' psychotic symptoms had been treated and to some extent stabilized prior to the group intervention. Topics discussed included friendship, personal economy, hygiene, understanding of mental health conditions—particularly psychotic symptoms—and the need for help. A meal was served at every group meeting to improve the social experience for the participants. Participants, family members, and professional caregivers described the intervention as helpful, and their experiences as positive, indicating that PMG is a feasible intervention for people with intellectual disabilities and psychosis.

Relapse Prevention and Crisis Management

A plan for crisis management should be provided for everyone with intellectual disabilities who are diagnosed with psychosis (Bakken et al., 2024). Such plans should include the person's specific early warning signs of a potential relapse. A crisis plan specifically describing symptoms of a potentially new psychotic episode has been considered important to reduce the risk of relapse (Birchwood et al., 2000). In the clinical sample mentioned above, 20 of 26 participants were provided with a plan for crisis management, which included early warning signs, contact information for the person's general practitioner and specialist mental health services, and a plan for adapted mental health nursing according to the person's current observed symptoms (Bakken et al., 2024). Providing a crisis management plan involving professional caregivers may be even more important for people with intellectual disabilities and psychosis than for other people with psychosis, as they usually have difficulties recognizing and reporting early warning signs.

Mental Health Nursing

This section emphasizes therapeutic skills in mental health nursing for people with intellectual disabilities and psychosis. Mental health nursing includes a range of different tasks. A competent mental health nurse has knowledge about mental health conditions, how symptoms and functional loss vary across people within diagnostic groups, and how mental health nursing interventions should be tailored to each person specifically. Additionally, the symptom burden experienced by people with psychosis may shift during episodes, throughout the day, and in acute phases, in minutes or even seconds. Monitoring these shifts requires the mental health nurse to have thorough knowledge about symptom presentation. This section addresses symptom observation, therapeutic communication, and creating good emotional climates.

Knowledge about symptom presentation is crucial, bearing in mind the problems of reporting inner mental states, especially for those diagnosed with psychosis (Bakken, 2021), even if they master communication about everyday matters in low-symptom phases. Such difficulties encompass both mentalization and introspection, especially in those with autism spectrum disorder in addition to intellectual disabilities, even for those with mild or moderate intellectual disabilities, which makes reporting on inner states difficult (Ribolsi et al., 2022; Robinson et al., 2017). They may not understand what is unusual and hence not tell others about it. Additionally, persons with intellectual disabilities, even those with borderline intellectual functioning, may not master the "language of illness" (Tuffrey-Wijne, 2013). They may not know how to describe physical pain, digestive problems, or other specific issues. See Chapter 2 for more about symptom presentation.

Observation of symptoms is one of the main tasks in mental health nursing for people with intellectual disabilities and psychosis (Bakken et al., 2008). People with psychosis, especially in acute phases, experience high levels of stress and anxiety. This phenomenon also includes people with intellectual disabilities (Bakken et al., 2007). Subjective experiences of anxiety may be difficult to report for persons with intellectual disabilities (Helverschou & Martinsen, 2011). However, signs of physiological arousal may be observed: rapid and superficial breathing, tachycardia, pupil dilation, pale facial skin, stiff body posture, and sweating . Additionally, dry mouth may be observed as frequent drinking and bathroom visits, or involuntary urination. Nausea may be hard to observe, but during strong anxiety reactions, vomiting may occur. During panic attacks, the following can be observed: restlessness, high motor activity, temper tantrums, attacks towards staff members or other people, running away, breaking items, and tearing down curtains. These behaviours may be interpreted as atypical anxiety reactions (Helverschou & Martinsen, 2011). Idiosyncratic behaviours can also be observed, such as ear flipping or repeatedly asking for specific items (Helverschou & Martinsen, 2011). Even experienced nursing staff working with people with the combination of intellectual disabilities and psychosis may have problems interpreting behaviour, especially in the acute phase of the illness (Bakken et al., 2008). Professionals must bear in mind that the use of behavioural equivalents to conventional symptoms will carry lower validity compared to person-reported symptoms (Bakken, 2021).

The main goal of therapeutic communication is providing symptom relief (Bakken et al., 2008). Therapeutic communication for people with intellectual disabilities and psychosis is usually effective when nurses perform task sustenance, attain joint attention, and provide meaningful responses and emotional support when communicating with the person. Reasonable adjustments for the person's cognitive impairments will aid in the development of alternative coping skills for negative symptoms, which have been found effective.

A review of mental health nursing interventions for people with intellectual disabilities and additional mental health conditions concludes that interventions used for the general population may be feasible for people with intellectual disabilities when adapted to their cognitive and adaptive level, and any additional neurocognitive impairments such as autism spectrum disorder (Bakken & Sageng, 2016). Bakken and Sageng underline the importance of understanding symptoms. An empirical study shows how difficult it may be to interpret the person's behaviour (Taua & Farrow, 2009). Observations revealed that staff had substantial problems differentiating between behaviour caused by a mental health condition and the person's regular behaviour caused by intellectual disabilities. For example, if a person appeared "noisy," one nurse might seclude him in his room, another might offer sedatives, while a third might do nothing.

Knowledge about personal communication style and possible idiosyncratic use of words or expressions is helpful for the nurse in order to understand the person (Bakken et al., 2008). Additionally, when communicating with people with intellectual disabilities and psychosis, it is found that the person may show considerably prolonged response times. Communication skills found to be useful in nursing for people in the general population, or for users with intellectual disabilities without psychosis, were also helpful when the person has both conditions. In the study by Bakken and colleagues, the participants showed significantly less disorganized behaviour and significantly more initiatives during interaction when staff members communicated effectively. They were not in an acute phase but still showing psychotic symptoms. This study elicited four main categories of effective communication skills that reduced psychotic symptoms: responding meaningfully, attention sustenance, task sustenance, and emotional support.

Responding meaningfully seemed to encourage initiatives in the participants but had the least impact on disorganized behaviour. Attention sustenance had a positive effect on disorganization. The results of the study also confirmed the importance of adjusting to the participant, as the communication partner seeks the person's attention area to achieve contact so the participant may focus on objects or persons. Task sustenance had the most prominent effect on disorganized behaviour in this sample. When task sustenance was used to help a strongly confused person who cannot perform the ongoing task, the person may become less frustrated and will experience the staff as both emotionally and practically supportive. Task sustenance helps the person to master an ongoing task, which may lead to fewer initiatives. Emotional support also seems to have strong effects on disorganized behaviour. When the staff provided emotional support in this study, the chance of organized behaviour in the participant was approximately 3:1. Bakken and colleagues found that providing emotional support instigates significantly more initiatives for interaction with staff compared to non-effective communication. Emotional support was operationalized as confirming feelings (validation), physical soothing, and mirroring (non-verbal validation) in the study conducted by Bakken and colleagues.

Emotional Climate

A good emotional climate, also described as ward atmosphere, is found to be favourable for people with severe mental illness who receive inpatient services, including people with intellectual disabilities (Bakken et al., 2012). The understanding of a good ward atmosphere as a potential therapeutic arena goes back about a hundred years. For people in the general population, two overlapping areas of research have dominated the literature on ward atmosphere: Gunderson's conceptualization of therapeutic components in mental health wards (Maree, 2001), and research on ward atmosphere in mental health inpatient units (Bell et al., 2018; Chester et al., 2015). Gunderson's therapeutic components are viewed as a valuable contribution to the creation of therapeutic milieus (Maree, 2001), and a number of studies have investigated their clinical applicability. The five components according to Gunderson are containment (provision of basic needs such as food, shelter, etc.), support (emphasizing experiences of well-being and feeling safe), structure (providing predictability), involvement (helping the person to improve social skills), and validation (Maree, 2001).

A qualitative study investigated the use of validation in mental health nursing for people with intellectual disabilities and additional mental health conditions in a specialized mental health inpatient setting (Bakken et al., 2017). Ten nurses/social educators and four individual therapists described the use of validation; each provided three short vignettes with clinical examples. The clinical examples support the view that interventions developed for people in the general population are also feasible for people with intellectual disabilities. Clinical implications support the use of validation as an important factor in mental health nursing for adults with intellectual disabilities, regardless of mental health diagnosis. Skills required include being capable of interpreting behavioural equivalents of symptoms, responding adequately to unusual utterances, and occasionally communicating predominantly nonverbally. The results from this study found nine categories of validation sorted into the two main factors of validation: acceptance and acknowledgement. Acceptance included adjusting interaction according to symptom load, adjusting staff expectations of task solving according to symptom load, and avoiding correction, directives during task solving, and reality checks. Acknowledgement included acknowledging emotions, individuality through special interests, requests or choices, and finally acknowledgement of adequate behaviour.

Community Services

Persons with multiple, complex needs including intellectual disabilities and severe mental health conditions usually need services from a wide range of health and social services, making coordination of care difficult (Dunn et al., 2020). Taking the high risk of relapse in psychosis into account, community care and follow-up should be emphasized (Franck et al., 2019). Regarding follow-up in community settings, assertive community treatment (ACT) has been found to be useful for people with intellectual disabilities and psychosis (Martin et al., 2005; Neijmeijer et al., 2018). Also, supervision and training of community caregivers may be necessary (Bakken et al., 2024). Collaborative meetings between different service levels will be important, as assessment and treatment conducted in specialist mental health services need to be integrated into community services.

Conclusive Remarks

The treatment and interventions presented in this chapter are predominantly developed for people in the general population and then adapted for people with intellectual disabilities. This is in line with the current understanding that mental health conditions in people with intellectual disabilities are the same phenomena as in people without intellectual disabilities. Adaptations for the most part include shorter sessions, bringing a support person into individual or group therapy, taking into account personal communication style/communication system in people who predominantly communicate non-verbally, using pictures or other visual support (for the whole range of intellectual disabilities), and having necessary knowledge about behavioural equivalents of psychotic and anxiety symptoms, especially in high symptom phases.

Research on mental health nursing for persons with intellectual disabilities and psychosis is still in its infancy. Some research indicates that interventions developed for the general population are feasible for people with intellectual disabilities and psychosis when properly adapted. But this topic is still understudied. There may be other interventions that also need individualized adaptations that have not yet been disclosed. More research on mental health nursing, especially regarding the effects of interventions, is needed and wanted.

References

Allott, K. A., Francey, S. M., & Velligan, D. I. (2013). Improving functional outcome using compensatory strategies in comorbid intellectual disability and psychosis: A case study. *American Journal of Psychiatric Rehabilitation, 16*(1), 50–65.

Andersen, C., Kolmos, A., Andersen, K., Sippel, V., & Stenager, E. (2017). Applying sensory modulation to mental health inpatient care to reduce seclusion and restraint: A case control study. *Nordic Journal of Psychiatry, 71*(7), 525–528.

Ashworth, S., Jansen, K., Bullock, L., & Mooney, P. (2017). Mind matters: A psychoeducation program for people with intellectual disabilities and co-morbid diagnoses of mental disorder. *Journal of Intellectual Disabilities and Offending Behaviour, 8*(1), 34–40.

Bakken, T. L. (2014). Psychosis and disorganized behaviour in adults with autism and intellectual disability: Case identification and staff-patient interaction. In V. B. Patel, V. R. Preedy, & C. R. Martin (Eds.), *Comprehensive guide to autism* (pp. 585–600). Springer Science.

Bakken, T. L. (2021). Et aapnere terapirom [A more open therapy room). *Utrednings- og behandlingssamtaler med personer med kognitiv funksjonshemming.* Fagbokforlaget.

Bakken, T. L., Askeland Hellerud, J. M., Kildahl, A. N., Solheim-Inderberg, A. M., Berge Helverschou, S., & Hove, O. (2024). Schizophrenia in Autistic people with intellectual disabilities. Treatment and interventions. *Journal of Autism and Developmental Disorders,* 1–11.

Bakken, T. L., Eilertsen, D. E., Smeby, N. A., & Martinsen, H. (2008). Effective communication related to psychotic disorganised behaviour in adults with intellectual disability and autism. *Nordic Journal of Nursing Research and Clinical Studies, 88*(28), 9–13.

Bakken, T. L., Friis, S., Lovoll, S., Smeby, N. A., & Martinsen, H. (2007). Behavioral disorganisation as an indicator of psychosis in adults with intellectual disability and autism. *Mental Health Aspects of Developmental Disabilities, 10*(2), 37–46.

Bakken, T. L., & Martinsen, H. (2013). Adults with intellectual disabilities and mental illness in psychiatric inpatient units. Empirical studies of patient characteristics and psychiatric diagnoses from 1996–2011. *International Journal of Developmental Disabilities, 59*(3), 179–190.

Bakken, T. L., Røssberg, J. I., & Friis, S. (2012). The use of the ward atmosphere scale for intellectually disabled psychiatric inpatients: A pilot study. *Advances in Mental Health and Intellectual Disabilities, 6*(5), 265–272.

Bakken, T.L. & Sageng, H. (2016). Mental health nursing of adults with intellectual disabilities and mental illness: A Review of Empirical Studies 1994–2013. *Archives of Psychiatric Nursing, 30*(2), 286–291.

Bakken, T. L., Sundby, I. L., & Klevmoen, G. H. (2017). Patients', family members', and professional carers' experiences of psychoeducational multifamily groups for participants with intellectual disabilities and mental illness. *Issues in Mental Health Nursing, 38*(2), 153–159.

Bell, N., Tonkin, M., Chester, V., & Craig, L. (2018). Adapting measures of social climate for use with people with intellectual disability in forensic settings. *Psychology, Crime & Law, 24*(4), 362–378.

Bighelli, I., Rodolico, A., García-Mieres, H., Pitschel-Walz, G., Hansen, W. P., Schneider-Thoma, J., Siafis, S., Wu, H., Wang, D., Salanti G., Furukawa, T. A., Barbui, C., & Leucht, S. (2021). Psychosocial and psychological interventions for relapse prevention in schizophrenia: A systematic review and network meta-analysis. *The Lancet Psychiatry, 8*(11), 969–980.

Birchwood, M., Spencer, E., & McGovern, D. (2000). Schizophrenia: Early warning signs. *Advances in Psychiatric Treatment, 6*(2), 93–101.

Chester, V., Mccathie, J., Quinn, M., Ryan, L., Popple, J., Loveridge, C., & Spall, J. (2015). Clinician experiences of administering the Essen Climate Evaluation Schema (EssenCES) in a forensic intellectual disability service. *Advances in Mental Health and Intellectual Disabilities, 9*(2), 70–78.

Chester, V., James, N., Rogers, I., Grace, J., & Alexander, R. (2020). Family experiences of psychiatric services for their relative with intellectual and developmental disabilities. In S. Bhaumik, & R. Alexander (Eds.), *Oxford textbook of the psychiatry of intellectual disability* (pp. 265–274). Oxford University Press.

Colvin, G., & Sheehan, M. R. (2014). *Managing the cycle of meltdown for students with autism.* Skyhorse Publishing.

Crowley, V., Rose, J., Smith, J., Hobster, K., & Ansell, E. (2008). Psycho-educational groups for people with a dual diagnosis of psychosis and mild intellectual disability: A preliminary study. *Journal of Intellectual Disabilities, 12*(1), 25–39.

Davis, E., Barnhill, L. J., & Saeed, S. A. (2008). Treatment models for treating patients with combined mental illness and developmental disability. *Psychiatric Quarterly, 79*, 205–223.

Dunn, K., Rydzewska, E., Fleming, M., & Cooper, S. A. (2020). Prevalence of mental health conditions, sensory impairments and physical disability in people with co-occurring intellectual disabilities and autism compared with other people: A cross-sectional total population study in Scotland. *British Medical Journal Open, 10*(4), Article e035280.

Franck, N., Bon, L., Dekerle, M., Plasse, J., Massoubre, C., Pommier, R., Legros-Lafarge, E., Jaafari, N., Guillard-Bouhet, N., Quilès, C., Couhet, G., Verdoux, H., Gouache, B., Martin, B., Cervello, S., Demily, C., & Dubreucq, J. (2019). Satisfaction and needs in serious mental illness and autism spectrum disorder: The REHABase psychosocial rehabilitation project. *Psychiatric Services, 70*(4), 316–323.

Gordon, P. C., Kauark, R. B. G., Costa, C. D. M., de Oliveira, M. O., Godinho, F. L. F., & Rocha, M. S. G. (2016). Clinical implications of the National Institute of Neurological Disorders and Stroke criteria for diagnosing psychosis in Parkinson's disease. *The Journal of Neuropsychiatry and Clinical Neurosciences, 28*(1), 26–31.

Guo, X., Zhai, J., Liu, Z., Fang, M., Wang, B., Wang, C., Hu, B., Sun, X., Lv, L., Lu, Z., Ma, C., He, X., Guo, T., Xie, S., Wu, R., Xue, Z., Chen, J., Twamley, E. W., Jin, H., & Zhao, J. (2010). Effect of antipsychotic medication alone vs combined with psychosocial intervention on outcomes of early-stage schizophrenia: A randomized, 1-year study. *Archives of General Psychiatry, 67*(9), 895–904.

Helverschou, S. B., & Martinsen, H. (2011). Anxiety in people diagnosed with autism and intellectual disability: Recognition and phenomenology. *Research in Autism Spectrum Disorders, 5*, 377–387.

Karlsen, K., Munkhaugen, E. K., Fossum, H. K., Bakken, T. L., & Kildahl, A. N. (2024). Mental health services for adults with intellectual disabilities: A qualitative study of patient characteristics, associated factors and consequent needs for adaptation in assessment and treatment. *Journal of Applied Research in Intellectual Disabilities, 38*(1), Article e13315.

Kerstein, L. H. (2008). *My sensory book: Working together to explore sensory issues and the big feelings they can cause: A workbook for parents, professionals, and children.* Aapc Publishing.

Maree, E. G. (2001). Hospital-based psychiatric nursing. In G. W. Stuart, & M. T. Laraia (Eds.), *Principles and practice of psychiatric nursing* (7th ed.). Mosby.

Martin, G., Costello, H., Leese, M., Slade, M., Bouras, N., Higgins, S., & Holt, G. (2005). An exploratory study of assertive community treatment for people with intellectual disability and psychiatric disorders: Conceptual, clinical, and service issues. *Journal of Intellectual Disability Research, 49*(7), 516–524.

McFarlane, W. R. (2016). Family interventions for schizophrenia and the psychoses: A review. *Family Process, 55*(3), 460–482.

Miguel, C. D. A. J., & Helen, K. (2011). Long-term mental health care for people with severe mental disorders.

Mulugeta, A., Suppiah, V., & Hyppönen, E. (2023). Schizophrenia and co-morbidity risk: Evidence from a data driven phenomewide association study. *Journal of Psychiatric Research, 162*, 1–10.

Neijmeijer, L. J., Didden, R., Nijman, H. L., & Kroon, H. (2018). Assertive community treatment for people with mild intellectual disability or borderline intellectual functioning and mental health problems or challenging behavior: State of the art and implementation in the Netherlands. *Journal of Policy and Practice in Intellectual Disabilities, 15*(4), 329–342.

Ribolsi, M., Nastro, F. F., Pelle, M., Medici, C., Sacchetto, S., Lisi, G., Riccioni, A., Siracusano, M., Mazzone, L., & Di Lorenzo, G. (2022). Recognizing psychosis in autism spectrum disorder. *Frontiers in Psychiatry, 13*, 768586.

Robinson, S., Howlin, P., & Russell, A. (2017). Personality traits, autobiographical memory and knowledge of self and others: A comparative study in young people with autism spectrum disorder. *Autism, 21*(3), 357–367.

Sommerstad, H. S., Kildahl, A. N., Munkhaugen, E. K., Karlsen, K., & Bakken, T. L. (2021). Experiences of ward atmosphere in inpatients with intellectual disability and mental illness: Clinical implications for mental health nursing. *International Journal of Developmental Disabilities, 67*(5), 339–348.

Taua, C., & Farrow, T. (2009). Negotiating complexities: An ethnographic study of intellectual disability and mental health nursing in New Zealand. *International Journal of Mental Health Nursing, 18*, 274–284.

Tuffrey-Wijne, I. (2013). A new model for breaking bad news to people with intellectual disabilities. *Palliative Medicine, 27*(1), 5–12.

van Os, J., & Kapur, S. (2009). Schizophrenia. *The Lancet, 374*(9690), 635–645.

Verhulst, I., MacLennan, K., Haffey, A., & Tavassoli, T. (2022). The perceived causal relations between sensory reactivity differences and anxiety symptoms in autistic adults. *Autism in Adulthood, 4*(3), 183–192.

8

Sensory Therapy

Charlotte Andersen

Abstract Sensory integration refers to the brain's ability to organize and process input from various sensory channels. It is the neurological mechanism that makes sense of sensory input from both inside our body and the environment. Persons with intellectual disabilities generally have problems processing sensory information. This problem may be aggravated by additional mental health conditions, causing everyday sensations to be experienced as perplexing or alarming. Sensory discomfort can lead to behaviour that challenges. By recognizing and addressing these underlying sensory integration difficulties, caregivers can tailor treatment plans to meet the sensory needs of each person, aiding their nervous systems in filtering and organizing sensory input effectively. This chapter includes a thorough description of sensory modulation disorder, sensory over- and under-responsivity, and an overview of evidence-based practices, illustrated by a case presentation.

C. Andersen (✉)
Fredericia, Denmark
e-mail: info@sanseprofilen.dk

T. L. Bakken (ed.), *Psychosis in Adolescents and Adults with Intellectual Disabilities*,
https://doi.org/10.1007/978-3-031-95318-7_8

Keywords Sensory modulation disorder · Sensory over-responsivity · Sensory under-responsivity · Sensory room · Sensory diet · Deep pressure stimulation

Understanding Sensory Modulation Disorder

Sensory integration refers to the brain's ability to organize and process input from various sensory channels, enabling adaptive responses as defined by Dr. A. Jean Ayres (1972). It is the neurological mechanism that helps us make sense of sensations from both our bodies and the environment, facilitating efficient interaction with our surroundings. However, persons with intellectual disabilities and severe mental health conditions often struggle with processing sensory information, finding even everyday sensations perplexing or alarming. Expressing their sensory discomfort can lead to behaviour that challenges, hindering effective communication with caregivers.

Sensory modulation disorder presents a significant challenge for persons with intellectual disabilities and psychosis, negatively affecting their performance and engagement in daily activities. These challenges can persist through adulthood, complicating the care process. Healthcare professionals may overlook or underestimate sensory integration dysfunction due to its complex nature, leading to misinterpretations of behaviour in persons with intellectual disabilities. Treatment methods, often language-centric, may not fully cater to their needs.

Miller and colleagues (2001) proposed the term "Sensory Processing Disorder" as an umbrella concept encompassing various sensory processing issues: Sensory Modulation Disorder, Sensory-Based Motor Disorder, and Sensory Discrimination Disorder

Sensory Modulation Disorder comprises three subtypes:

- Sensory over-responsivity
- Sensory under-responsivity
- Sensory seeking

Subtypes of Sensory-Based Motor Disorder include:

- Dyspraxia
- Postural disorder

Sensory Discrimination Disorder encompasses subtypes such as:

- Visual
- Auditory
- Tactile
- Gustatory (taste)
- Olfactory (smell)
- Vestibular (movement in space)
- Proprioceptive (awareness of body position and movement)
- Interoception (sensing internal body signals)

Sensory Over-Responsivity

Persons exhibiting over-responsivity may easily feel overwhelmed by sensory stimuli encountered in daily life, including sounds, smells, visual movements, and touch. These experiences can accumulate throughout the day, leading to fatigue or challenging behaviours. Since verbal communication may be challenging for those with intellectual disabilities and psychosis, professional caregivers play a crucial role in understanding and supporting these persons. Balancing exposure to sensory stimuli with appropriate strategies to limit intensity or duration is essential for maintaining engagement without overwhelming them. Flexibility in adjusting plans is often necessary to achieve this balance.

Sensory Under-Responsivity

Conversely, some persons may struggle to notice environmental sensations due to under-responsivity. They may be unaware of objects, changes in terrain, or variations in temperature, and typically require increased sensory input throughout the day. It is important to note that people can experience both over- and under-responsivity simultaneously, depending on the senses involved and the context. When creating a sensory plan, each sense and its context should be carefully considered.

Sensory Seeking

Persons with a sensory seeking profile actively pursue sensory stimulation throughout the day. However, their intense sensory cravings may lead to disruptive behaviours, such as touching others or objects excessively. While they may seem to require constant stimulation, excessive input can lead to dysregulation, affecting impulse control, focus, and behaviour.

Dyspraxia

Dyspraxia, a sensory-based motor disorder, affects movement and coordination skills, including tasks requiring balance or fine motor skills. Symptoms can vary between persons and may affect daily activities, social functioning, and emotional regulation. Routine tasks may be particularly challenging for these persons.

Postural Disorder

Persons with postural disorder exhibit poor core strength and endurance, leading to inefficient movement and low body awareness. They may demonstrate cautious or reluctant movement, preferring sedentary activities. Signs include poor muscle coordination, fatigue, and difficulty maintaining stable positions.

Sensory Discrimination Disorder

Sensory discrimination disorder can affect various senses, making it challenging to discern sensory information accurately. For example, difficulties may arise in distinguishing sounds in a noisy environment or navigating crowded spaces. Discrimination issues involving the vestibular system can cause disorientation in situations like revolving doors. Similarly, challenges in interception may lead to confusion regarding bodily signals, such as hunger or fatigue (Ayres, 1971).

Methods and Modalities

Caregivers supporting people with intellectual disabilities and psychosis should consider that the cognitive demands might exceed the person's capacity. Overwhelming demands can lead to confusion and anxiety. Using a metaphorical "house" model, where the central nervous system forms the foundation and higher cognitive functions represent the top levels, caregivers must address sensory modulation issues at the foundation level before progressing to higher cognitive functions (Williams & Shellenberger, 1996).

Evidence-Based Practice: Sensory-Based Modalities

Based on available evidence, sensory interventions appear to yield favourable social, emotional, and cognitive outcomes for persons living with intellectual disabilities (Humpheson, 2024; Hylkema & Vlaskamp, 2009). Key aspects of these interventions include the judicious application of sensory stimuli, the involvement of skilled facilitators, and adherence to more rigorous intervention schedules. Notable improvements include decreases in behaviour that challenges, and stress levels, alongside enhancements in engagement, attention, and communication skills. From the data, three overarching themes have surfaced, underscoring pivotal elements of sensory interventions for this population: tailoring sensory stimuli to person needs, involvement of trained sensory integration therapists and caregivers as facilitators, and the importance of extended intervention periods with increased frequency (Bundy et al., 2002).

People with intellectual disabilities who are in a psychotic state may appear confused, disorganized, and have impaired communication, along with significant problems in task-solving (Bakken et al., 2007). They may also exhibit agitation, aggression, and stress, and have difficulties regulating basic needs such as sleep, rest, and food. Therefore, support for regulation is necessary. Sensory therapy has been found to be both effective and feasible for persons with cognitive impairments (Green et al., 2020; Justice et al., 2021), and, alongside medication, may be a highly beneficial intervention.

A case may illustrate how different sensory-based modalities can be combined. "John," in his mid-twenties, arrived at a specialized mental health inpatient unit for adults with intellectual disabilities (Bakken & Høidal, 2019), where he stayed for more than six months. Upon arrival, he appeared completely fragmented and experienced several panic attacks daily. For weeks, he slept only a couple of hours each night. Diagnostic assessment concluded with the following diagnoses: mild intellectual disabilities, psychosis, and autistic traits. The inpatient unit had a large bathtub, and John became accustomed to using it every day. When he was stressed out and displayed high levels of anxiety, he could stay in the bathtub for several hours. He also used a weighted blanket, choosing for himself when and how long to use the blanket or the bathtub. He told the staff that staying in water or under a weighted blanket was "much better than the pills." He continued to use baths and a weighted blanket after being discharged from the inpatient unit.

Sensory Rooms

Personalizing sensory strategies and interventions is paramount. Different persons may exhibit over-responsiveness to some senses and under-responsiveness to others. Therefore, it is essential to tailor a sensory plan to meet the client's specific sensory, medical, therapeutic needs, and goals. A multi-modal approach should be employed. Many people can benefit from utilizing a sensory room equipped with calming modalities such as a ball mattress, weighted blankets, nature sounds and images, and aromatherapy. A Sensory room offers a much-needed and soothing sensory respite from accumulated overload or emotional stress.

Sensory Rooms in Mental Health Practice

Andersen and colleagues (2017) showed the efficacy of integrating a sensory room into inpatient mental health care, illustrating a significant reduction in the requirement for restraint and forced medication among people with psychosis. Employing the sensory profile assessment, the sensory room was utilized in a client-centred manner to identify and cater to the sensory needs of users. This approach, primarily aimed at preventing restraint, also served to soothe distressed people experiencing psychosis or withdrawal symptoms.

Sensory Rooms and Verbal Communication Disorders

Consideration should be given to the impact of receptive/expressive language disorders and auditory processing conditions to effectively engage in treatment. People with both intellectual disabilities and psychosis tend to communicate sparsely during high-symptom phases, even those who normally express themselves adequately (Bakken et al., 2007). Since treatment approaches toward psychosis for adolescents and adults heavily rely on language processing, we may inadvertently choose a treatment modality that is least accessible to people with intellectual disabilities. A significant portion of people with intellectual disabilities, who develop psychosis, encounter substantial challenges in processing verbal information.

By utilizing a sensory room, we have the opportunity to make every aspect of the treatment process multi-modal, incorporating verbal, visual, movement, kinaesthetic, and musical elements. This approach not only fosters a greater integration of the treatment experience, but also helps people feel more competent, motivated, engaged, and understood throughout their journey in therapy.

Sensory Rooms and Autism

People with autism spectrum disorder may experience sensitivity to clothing, loud sounds, or certain smells, leading to sensory overload and resulting behaviours such as refusing to wear certain clothes, covering their ears, or engaging in repetitive movements (Werkman et al., 2023). Accommodating or regulating these sensory issues can help ease discomfort and support emotional regulation. Sensory rooms can be specifically designed to control sensory experiences, providing a calming environment and accommodating persons with sensory sensitivities.

Strategies may include earplugs, headphones, fidget toys, weighted blankets, soft textures, light covers, sunglasses, and other sensory tools, as well as soft lighting, calming paint colours, and adjustable seating. Multisensory environments or sensory rooms have been found to be effective in helping people with autism better control their emotions, promoting autonomy and a sense of control. People with autism often feel powerless due to sensory processing issues, and having access to a sensory room can help reduce anxiety by providing a safe space to down regulate stress and cope with sensory challenges. Additionally, sensory rooms can help manage challenging behaviours by providing a supportive and calming environment. Redirecting persons experiencing sensory overload to a sensory room can quickly reduce their distress and allow them to refocus their attention.

Sensory "Diet"

Coined by Wilbarger (1995) the term "sensory diet" refers to a personalized daily routine designed to proactively address safety and sensory needs. It encompasses a range of strategies readily accessible throughout the day. For instance, this might include personalized essential oils, a rubber ball for foot rolling, breathing exercises using a straw, tactile fidgets, mandala colouring, and more. These sensory elements should be readily available throughout the day, including when the person is away from home.

The Powerhouses and Deep Pressure

The primary senses—tactile, vestibular, and proprioception—are fundamental components of our sensory foundation. While we often address these sensory systems personally, they are intricately intertwined and can influence each other in various ways.

Referred to as the "powerhouses," the primary senses play a crucial role as their input often is perceived as calming and capable of reducing anxiety and dysregulation. Light tactile stimuli typically trigger alertness, whereas deep pressure touch stimulation tends to induce feelings of calmness, grounding, and self-awareness. Proprioception, *the* ability to determine the position of own body parts, utilized therapeutically, involves selecting activities that engage and stimulate the proprioceptive system, such as walking, lifting, pulling, pushing, and isometric exercises.

The vestibular system can exhibit both under-responsiveness and over-responsiveness. Depending on the person's response to vestibular stimuli, intervention strategies should be carefully selected. For persons with under-responsive vestibular systems, interventions aimed at increasing input are chosen, while for those with over-responsive systems, interventions must be applied with great caution.

Weighted Modalities

A weighted modality is a type of sensory-based intervention that offers both tactile and proprioceptive input (Champagne et al., 2015; Chen et al., 2013; Mullen et al., 2008). This intervention comes in various forms and styles, including integrated options like chair cushions or pillows, as well as standalone items such as weighted blankets, vests, large floor mats, or mattress toppers. Hylkema and Vlaskamp (2009) found that the use of weighted blankets significantly improved sleep among persons with intellectual disabilities.

The purpose of a weighted modality is to provide people with deep proprioceptive and tactile sensory input. People with intellectual and/or mental psychosis experience that weighted modalities lead to improvements in sleep quality, heightened body awareness, increased attention span, and enhanced regulation of emotions (Andersen et al., 2017; Justice et al., 2021; Werkman et al., 2023). For persons living with intellectual disabilities and psychosis, utilizing a weighted modality can promote a stronger sense of self and feelings of stability and grounding. This intervention may also assist persons in coping with distressing experiences such as confusion or psychotic episodes.

Arousal

To effectively engage in activities and respond adaptively to sensory input, the arousal level must be appropriately balanced. The Yerkes-Dodson model (1908) shows that when arousal levels are excessively high, users might experience feelings of alarm or anxiety, potentially leading to sensory overload. Conversely, when arousal levels are too low, clients may struggle with motivation and concentration, consequently affecting their engagement and performance. Achieving the optimal arousal level is crucial (Fig. 8.1).

Persons with intellectual disabilities often contend with low arousal levels, which may prompt sensory self-stimulation behaviours. At

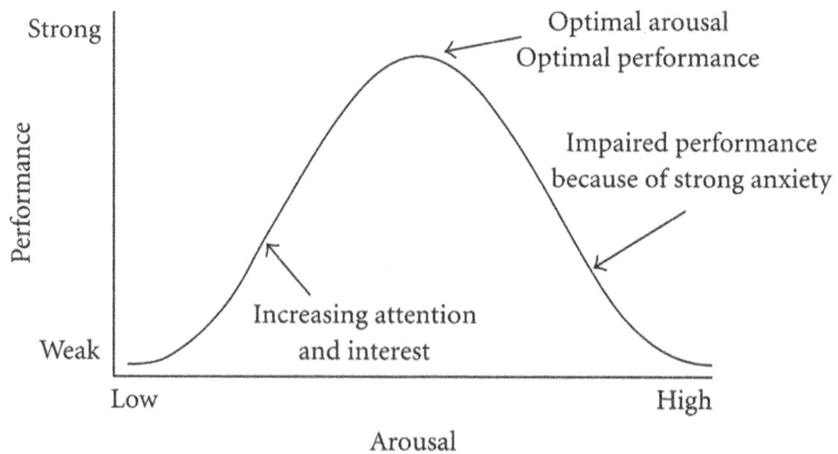

Fig. 8.1 The Yerkes-Dodson's model of arousal (1908)

times, caregivers may view sexual self-stimulation as a challenging behaviour, particularly when it becomes excessive or results in tissue damage. However, these extreme manifestations of self-stimulation often stem from underlying arousal issues. By addressing the root cause of arousal dysregulation, persons may experience reduced reliance on self-stimulation behaviours.

Conclusive Remarks

Persons with intellectual disabilities often grapple with either too low or too high levels of arousal, with some experiencing low arousal during the day and heightened arousal before bedtime. People with both intellectual disabilities and psychosis are known to exhibit severe dysfunctional regulation, especially during phases with high symptom load. Sensory therapy may be a feasible intervention, as part of a multi-modal treatment program.

References

Andersen, C., Kolmos, A., Andersen, K., Sippel, V., & Stenager, E. (2017). Applying sensory modulation to mental health inpatient care to reduce seclusion and restraint: A case control study. *Nordic Journal of Psychiatry, 71*(7), 525–528.

Ayres, A. J. (1971). Characteristics of types of sensory integrative dysfunction. *American Journal of Occupational Therapy, 25*, 329–334.

Ayres, A. J. (1972). *Sensory integration and learning disorders*. Western Psychological Services.

Bakken, T. L., Friis, S., Lovoll, S., Smeby, N. A., & Martinsen, H. (2007). Behavioral disorganisation as an indicator of psychosis in adults with intellectual disability and autism. *Mental Health Aspects of Developmental Disabilities, 10*(2), 37–46.

Bakken, T. L., & Høidal, S. H. (2019). Specialized psychiatric services: Patient characteristics, referral practice and length of stay in a representative clinical sample 2010–2016. *International Journal of Developmental Disabilities, 65*(4), 277–284.

Bundy, A., Lane, S., & Murray, E. (2002). *Sensory integration: Theory and practice*. F.A. Davis Company.

Champagne, T., Mullen, B., Dickson, D., & Krishnamurty, S. (2015). Evaluating the safety and effectiveness of the weighted blanket with adults during an inpatient mental health hospitalization. *Occupational Therapy in Mental Health, 31*(3), 211–233. https://doi.org/10.1080/0164212X.2015.1066220.

Chen, H. Y., Yang, H., Chi, H. J., & Chen, H. M. (2013). Physiological effects of deep touch pressure on anxiety alleviation: The weighted blanket approach. *Journal of Medical and Biological Engineering, 33*(5), 463–470.

Green, L., Willis, E., Ziev, N., Oliveira, D., Kornblau, B., & Robertson, S. (2020). The impact of weighted blankets on the sleep and sensory experiences of autistic adults. *American Journal of Occupational Therapy, 74*(S1), NA–NA.

Humpheson, J. (2024). Sensory approaches for adults with severe or profound and multiple learning disabilities: A systematic literature review. *British Journal of Occupational Therapy, 87*(3), 129–142.

Hylkema, T., & Vlaskamp, C. (2009). Significant improvement in sleep in people with intellectual disabilities living in residential settings by non-pharmaceutical interventions. *Journal of Intellectual Disability Research, 53*(8), 695–703.

Justice, H., Haines, D., & Wright, J. (2021). Occupational therapy for adults with intellectual disabilities and sensory processing challenges: A Delphi study exploring practice within acute assessment and treatment units. *Irish Journal of Occupational Therapy, 49*(1), 28–35.

Miller, L. J., Reisman, J. E., McIntosh, D. N., & Simon, J. (2001). An ecological model of sensory modulation: Performance of children with fragile X syndrome, autistic disorder, ADHD, and sensory modulation dysfunction. In S. S. Roley (Eds.), *Understanding the nature of sensory integration with diverse populations*.

Mullen, B., Champagne, T., Krishnamurty, S., Dickson, D., & Gao, R. X. (2008). Exploring the safety and therapeutic effects of deep pressure stimulation using a weighted blanket. *Occupational Therapy in Mental Health, 24*(1), 65–89.

Werkman, M. F., Landsman, J. A., Fokkens, A. S., Dijkxhoorn, Y. M., van Berckelaer-Onnes, I. A., Begeer, S., & Reijneveld, S. A. (2023). The impact of the presence of intellectual disabilities on sensory processing and behavioral outcomes among individuals with autism spectrum disorders: A systematic review. *Review Journal of Autism and Developmental Disorders, 10*(3), 422–440.

Wilbarger, P. (1995). The sensory diet: Activity programs based on sensory processing theory. *American Occupational Therapy Association, 18*(2), 1–3.

Williams, M. S., & Shellenberger S. (1996). *How does your engine run? Leader's guide to the alert program for self-regulation.* TherapyWorks.

Yerkes, R. M., & Dodson, J. D. (1908). The relation of strength of stimulus to rapidity of habit-formation. *Journal of Comparative Neurology and Psychology, 18*(5), 459–482.

9

The Users' and the Families' Perspectives

Trine Lise Bakken

Abstract Knowledge about the opinions and experiences of users and their families regarding mental health services for people with intellectual disabilities is generally limited. Experiences from these services, and their everyday life with psychosis, for those with both intellectual disabilities and psychosis, are very sparse. Hence, this chapter will also refer to studies including individuals with psychosis in the general population, or individuals with intellectual disabilities and mental health conditions in general, in addition to the experiences of their families.

Keywords User experiences · Family experiences

T. L. Bakken (✉)
Oslo University Hospital, Oslo, Norway
e-mail: uxtlba@ous-hf.no

T. L. Bakken (ed.), *Psychosis in Adolescents and Adults with Intellectual Disabilities*,
https://doi.org/10.1007/978-3-031-95318-7_9

The User's Perspectives

During the last decade, patient-reported outcome measures (PROM) have been found to be more clinically relevant compared to measures reported by health professionals (Mercieca-Bebber et al., 2017). Several papers, which have included informants with intellectual disabilities, report findings in line with this new approach in clinical research. A discrepancy between user-reported symptoms and symptoms reported by family members or professional caregivers highlights the need for user participation for persons with intellectual disabilities, both during assessment and especially during decision-making (Rose, 2013). A study on anger and intellectual disabilities reported that people with mild and moderate intellectual disabilities report more emotions and mental health issues, whereas professional caregivers reported more behaviour that challenges (Rose, 2013). This discrepancy should influence both clinical practice and research in the area of mental health in people with intellectual disabilities.

Over the last decades, former and present users of mental health services in the general population have shared their experiences about living with psychosis (Walsh et al., 2016). Walsh and colleagues identified five major themes through a systematic review on what it is like to live with psychosis: the experience of symptoms, the process of acceptance, personal relationships, treatment experiences, and spiritual practices and faith. This is an important study, as most psychosis research has focused on phenomenology, especially core symptoms, prevalence and incidence, antipsychotic treatment, and follow-up. Regarding symptoms, hallucinations were experienced as frightening, confusing, and exhausting. In addition, disorientation appeared as frightening. Furthermore, "loss of self" and "loss of identity" were mentioned as important. Taken together, it is likely that these lived experiences are also relevant for people with intellectual disabilities who are diagnosed with psychosis, although they have a reduced capacity to report such symptoms and experiences.

A Scandinavian qualitative study interviewed 24 adults with psychosis, who were provided multimodal treatment including antipsychotic medication, and all of them had many years of contact with mental health services, both outpatient and inpatient (Møllerhøj et al., 2020). The participants described a variety of challenges in everyday functioning, especially emphasizing not being part of the workforce. They rated their mental and physical well-being as good. The study underlines that recovery for persons with psychosis is a long-lasting process. The participants emphasized the importance of robust relationships with mental health professionals, therapeutic conversations, antipsychotic medications, and support from relatives during recovery (Møllerhøj et al., 2020).

The results from the Møllerhøj study are in line with a Norwegian study on experiences from inpatient stays in specialized mental health services for people with intellectual disabilities (Sommerstad et al., 2021). The study interviewed 10 adolescents and adults with intellectual disabilities about their views on ward atmosphere. Three of the participants were diagnosed with psychosis (Sommerstad et al., 2021). The participants' experience of their relationships with ward staff was found to be the most important factor regarding their experiences of inpatient stay. Additionally, feeling safe, contained, and validated were rated as important aspects. That relationships with therapists are the most important outcome was also found in a study on individual therapy for people with intellectual disabilities and depression (Knight et al., 2019). The Knight study used self-reported patient outcomes.

An English qualitative study is one of only a handful of articles on user experiences of having co-morbid intellectual disabilities and psychosis (Robinson et al., 2016). Robinson and colleagues explored the experiences and views of five adults with mild intellectual disabilities and psychosis in community settings. They were asked about their experiences of having intellectual disabilities and an additional psychosis, and of the services they were provided. The participants seemed to be confused about their diagnoses and symptoms and communicated less insight than expected by the researchers. They were more concerned about understanding themselves and having individual and specific needs. However, they appreciated the support they received from mental health professionals and were able to describe the practical and emotional support they needed. These findings contradict the Swedish study, where the participants were well-informed about their conditions. It may be that people with intellectual disabilities need more thorough education about mental health issues compared to the general population (Crowley et al., 2008).

An Australian qualitative study included six adults with intellectual disabilities and additional mental health conditions (Weise et al., 2018). The participants were interviewed about their opinions on mental health services for people with intellectual disabilities, particularly their positive and negative experiences and suggestions for improvements. The findings are in line with other research cited in this chapter, and also in Chapter 7, underlining the importance of communication skills in mental health professionals. Other important topics were working with a person's support network and increasing user participation, especially in the roles of educators and peer workers. The participants also emphasized the importance of respect for the users.

A review investigated the views and experiences of adults with intellectual disabilities accessing digital mental health interventions (MacHale et al., 2023). The study concludes that new technology has the potential to be a helpful complement to regular mental health services for people with intellectual disabilities. The five included studies were qualitative, involving adults with intellectual disabilities and additional mental health conditions. Most of the participants were positive about digital mental health interventions. An interesting finding was that the participants viewed their contact with a therapist, even though the therapist was an avatar, as a "therapeutic relationship." Another interesting finding was that, in addition to task-oriented support, the participants also appreciated support to navigate their computers and to regulate stress triggered by the cognitive and emotional challenge of accessing technology. However, the participants emphasized that they did not want to replace their regular therapist with a computer.

Five adults with intellectual disabilities and mental health conditions, two of whom were diagnosed with psychosis, participated in a Norwegian book project (Bakken, 2021). The participants had recovered from acute phases and were living in around-the-clock staffed group homes. The book was about clinical interviews and psychotherapy. Both former users and present therapists participated and shared their opinions and experiences about assessment and therapy. One of the participants had recovered almost completely from psychosis but experienced symptoms occasionally, especially in stressful situations like being with unknown staff. For him, as well as the four other participants in this project, relationships with therapists and staff members were paramount and emphasized as the most important aspect of mental health inpatient services. This participant had a robust working alliance with his psychologist and was proud of the work he did during sessions with her: "Yes, I did well. It was a good feeling. Yes, I had to work hard. I get some sort of reward after the hard work. I have a good life now. I can enjoy my bachelorhood."

Trust was another topic mentioned. One of the participants emphasized how she trusted her therapist by daring to disagree: "I dared to disagree with her. Very much so. I dared to be a little bit angry. It was safe to disagree. It did not hurt to disagree." Another participant spoke about the head of the group home where he lives: "He told me something that I have never heard before. He said that he had to show me that he trusted me, by letting me go with him in his car. I didn't know that he thought like that. He had to do this so that I could accept him."

The five participants agreed about assessments. They did not like this part of mental health services. One said: "It was some tests. It was a bit difficult. The thing with questions like that is difficult. I don't like it." Another participant with psychosis had been through many assessments, which she did not like. She was in remission when she was interviewed for the project. She emphasized that she needed information about why it is important to go through tests and questions about her mental state: "You explained why I have to do it. Because I hate it. You said to me 'I think you need more help where you live.' Then I understood that you do it because you want to help. The assessment helped me to understand that I need more help."

The participant above, who hates assessment, was eager to know more about how psychotic symptoms impact her brain. Here is an excerpt from a transcript from therapy (P is the user; T is the therapist):

- P: Is the brain very tired after being psychotic? I am still on the couch. I am tired from resting, but I cannot do anything else. It is also very tiresome to think.

- T: You describe fatigue (another word for being very tired) very well. Your brain is exhausted from being very stressed by the psychotic symptoms. Psychosis is very tough for the brain.
- P: I want to get well very soon. I am afraid that I have to be like this forever. Do you think I should push myself to do more?
- T: No, I do not think you should push yourself to do more. Rest treatment might be good for you. What about using the tub? Or use your headphones to listen to music. It could help your brain to be less distressed. You will not be like this forever

The Family Experiences

Family members of persons with intellectual disabilities and additional mental health conditions are found to experience high-stress levels (Syeda et al., 2011), especially for families that care for their sons or daughters at home. A Canadian study found that in a group of 29 families, almost 60% were facing an upcoming crisis (Syeda et al., 2011). Moreover, in more than half of the families, one of the parents had to quit their job or work less, which in turn negatively affected the family economy.

Two Norwegian studies investigated the family experiences of mental health services for adults with intellectual disabilities and mental health conditions (Matheussen et al., 2020; Sommerstad et al., 2024). Three Norwegian mothers of adult offspring with cognitive impairments and psychosis participated in a book project on mental health nursing in mental health services for people with intellectual disabilities (Matheussen et al., 2020). They knew each other well from a psychoeducational group for mothers. The three mothers had 30, 20, and 15 years of experience, respectively, with mental health services, habilitation services, and community services. They emphasized that "well-educated professionals," such as psychologists and social pedagogues, were too concerned with behaviour that challenges. They felt that the emphasis on behaviour problems "blocked" the understanding of the inner life of their offspring: "We need professionals who can help us maintain hope. Although it is difficult, we need to be told about people who have recovered from mental ill health." Another important topic for the mothers was reading case files. From their experiences, reading case files could be overwhelming: "All the nasty stuff about my son in the hospital records—it is a hard read for me." The last main topic for the mothers was therapeutic communication: "People with intellectual disabilities are often unable to express how they feel, what they think, or what they want, especially in bad times with heavy symptoms. They need help to express themselves."

Family members of eight adults in mental health services for people with intellectual disabilities participated in a qualitative survey on family experiences (Sommerstad et al., 2024). The family members emphasized that staff members should have expertise about people with co-morbid intellectual disabilities and severe mental health conditions, and hence have the required communication skills. Trust in staff for the participants was important for family members in order to feel safe, and an extra effort may be necessary to build such trust among the families. Furthermore, the availability of staff was important: "We have been involved all the way. The cooperation with staff members and the psychologist worked well. They listened to me". Staff members being available to answer phone calls and frequent contact points were emphasized by the participants as facilitating involvement and collaboration between the families and the services.

Another article was written in collaboration between mental health professionals and a mother of a young man, "Harald," who was diagnosed with cognitive impairments and psychosis (Bakken et al., 2015). The aim of the article was to illuminate that long-lasting collaboration between the family, specialist mental health services, and community services is paramount for users with multiple, complex needs, including psychosis and intellectual disabilities. Harald experienced severe loss of adaptive skills since adolescence. He was several times referred to habilitation services and specialist mental health services without a proper explanation for his problems. Harald's mother asked the local mental health services for a second opinion from another health region, which was accepted after several attempts. A new group of helpers was established, including local mental health services (both inpatient and outpatient services), habilitation services, and local community services.

Two therapists from a larger hospital participated in the group for six years. The main therapist from the larger hospital had regular telephone contact with Harald's mother throughout the entire course. Harald's mother had been an instigator for proper assessment and treatment since Harald's first signs of a possible mental health condition. She told me several times about being perceived and characterized as "troublesome," "overinvolved," "a hindrance to Harald's development," and other less beneficial characteristics. However, without his mother, Harald would probably not have been referred for a second opinion, and hence not recovered from psychosis.

Conclusive Remarks

The articles cited in this chapter have in common that there are few participants, and therefore a limited body of research. Hence, no firm conclusions can be drawn, except for the need for more research on user experiences. In spite of this, experiences and opinions shared by the users and their close family members may enlighten clinical practice. For example, regarding mental health nursing, user participation should technically be easy to achieve, as the nursing staff in mental health institutions, as well as in community care, are the professionals who spend most of the time with the users. However, people with intellectual disabilities still have generally limited impact on interventions in mental health and community services. Important insights from both users and their families underline that the professional relationships between the patients and their families may be as valuable for them as the use of specific interventions. These relationships require time, as for the mother quoted above, who worked with the therapeutic team over a 6-year period.

References

Bakken, T. L. (2021). *Et aapnere terapirom [A more open therapy room]*. Fagbokforlaget.

Bakken, T. L., Heien, G., Neset, B., & Harald's mother. (2015). Mental health services for persons with psychosis, autism, and aberrant behaviour – multidisciplinary and interagency collaboration [Psykisk helsearbeid for mennesker med psykose, autisme og utfordrende atferd – tverrfaglig og tverretatlig samarbeid]. *Fontene.no*.

Crowley, V., Rose, J., Smith, J., Hobster, K., & Ansell, E. (2008). Psycho—educational groups for people with a dual diagnosis of psychosis and mild intellectual disability: A preliminary study. *Journal of Intellectual Disabilities, 12*(1), 25–39.

Knight, R., Jahoda, A., Scott, K., Sanger, K., Knowles, D., Dagnan, D., Hastings, R. P., Appleton, K., Cooper, S.-A., Melville, C., Jones, R., Williams, C., & Hatton, C. (2019). Getting into it: People with intellectual disabilities' experiences and views of behavioural activation and guided self-help for depression. *Journal of Applied Research in Intellectual Disabilities, 32,* 819–830.

MacHale, R., French, C., & McGuire, B. (2023). The experiences and views of adults with intellectual disabilities accessing digital mental health interventions: A qualitative systematic review and thematic synthesis. *Journal of Applied Research in Intellectual Disabilities, 36*(3), 448–457.

Matheussen, I., Farnes, E., Boe, V. N., & Bakken T. L. (2020). Family experiences and co-operation with mental health staff members [Familiens erfaringer og samarbeid med miljøterapeuter]. In T. L. Bakken (Eds.), *Handbook of mental health nursing. For children and adults with intellectual and developmental disorders [Håndbok i miljøterapi. Til barn og voksne med kognitiv funksjonshemming]* (pp. 215–226). Fagbokforlaget.

Mercieca-Bebber, R., Friedlander, M., Calvert, M., Stockler, M., Kyte, D., Kok, P. S., & King, M. T. (2017). A systematic evaluation of compliance and reporting of patient-reported outcome endpoints in ovarian cancer randomised controlled trials: Implications for generalisability and clinical practice. *Journal of Patient-Reported Outcomes, 1,* 1–10.

Møllerhøj, J., Os Stølan, L., Erdner, A., Hedberg, B., Stahl, K., Riise, J., Jedenius, E., & Rise, M. B. (2020). "I live, I don't work, but I live a very normal life"—A qualitative interview study of Scandinavian user experiences of schizophrenia, antipsychotic medication, and personal recovery processes. *Perspectives in Psychiatric Care, 56*(2).

Robinson, L., Escopri, N., Stenfert, B., Kroese, & Rose, J. (2016). The subjective experience of adults with intellectual disabilities who have mental health problems within community settings. *Advances in Mental Health and Intellectual Disabilities, 10*(2), 106–115.

Rose, J. (2013). A preliminary investigation into the influence of therapist experience on the outcome of individual anger interventions for people with intellectual disabilities. *Behavioural and Cognitive Psychotherapy, 41*(4), 470–478.

Sommerstad, H. S., Kildahl, A. N., Augustin, M., & Bakken, T. L. (2024). Ward atmosphere for inpatients with intellectual disability and mental illness: family members' perceptions and experience. *International Journal of Developmental Disabilities,* 1–9.

Sommerstad, H. S., Kildahl, A. N., Munkhaugen, E. K., Karlsen, K., & Bakken, T. L. (2021). Experiences of ward atmosphere in inpatients with intellectual disability and mental illness: Clinical implications for mental health nursing. *International Journal of Developmental Disabilities, 67*(5), 339–348.

Syeda, M., Weiss, J., & Lunsky, Y. (2011). Experiences of families of individuals with intellectual disability and psychiatric disorder. *Journal on Developmental Disabilities, 17*(2), 64–68.

Walsh, J., Hochbrueckner, R., Corcoran, J., & Spence, R. (2016). The lived experience of schizophrenia: A systematic review and meta-synthesis. *Social Work in Mental Health, 14*(6), 607–624.

Weise, J., Fisher, K. R., Whittle, E., & Trollor, J. N. (2018). What can the experiences of people with an intellectual disability tell us about the desirable attributes of a mental health professional? *Journal of Mental Health Research in Intellectual Disabilities, 11*(3), 183–202.

Index

T. L. Bakken (ed.), *Psychosis in Adolescents and Adults with Intellectual Disabilities*, https://doi.org/10.1007/978-3-031-95318-7

N

O

P

R

S

T

The manufacturer's authorised representative in the EU is Springer Nature Customer Service Centre GmbH, Europaplatz 3, 69115 Heidelberg, Germany. If you have any concerns regarding our products, please contact ProductSafety@springernature.com

Printed and bound by CPI Group (UK) Ltd, Croydon, CR0 4YY

12/06/2026

02136105-0001